HOW TO USE
INDEX MEDICUS
AND
EXCERPTA MEDICA

Forthcoming titles in the Information Sources in the Medical Sciences series by Barry Strickland-Hodge

How to use Biological Abstracts, Chemical Abstracts and Psychological Abstracts

How to Search the Medical Sources

HOW TO USE
INDEX MEDICUS
AND
EXCERPTA MEDICA

Dr. Barry Strickland-Hodge

Director, Medical Information Research Unit,
School of Library and Information Studies
Leeds Polytechnic
and
Managing Director,
Medical Information Technology
and Training Ltd

Gower

© Barry Stickland-Hodge, 1986

All rights reserved. No part of this publication may be reproduced, stored in a retrieval system, or transmitted in any form or by any means, electronic, mechanical, photocopying, recording or otherwise without the prior permission of Gower Publishing Company Limited.

Published by

Gower Publishing Company Limited,
Gower House,
Croft Road,
Aldershot,
Hants GU11 3HR
England

Gower Publishing Company,
Old Post Road
Brookfield
Vermont 05036
U.S.A.

British Library Cataloguing in Publication Data

Strickland-Hodge, B.
   How to use Index medicus and Excerpta medica. — (Information sources in the medical sciences; 1)
   1. Index medicus   2. Excerpta medica
   3. Medicine — Abstracting and indexing
   I. Title   II. Series
   025'.0667   R119

ISBN: 0 566 03532 4

Typeset in Great Britain by Action Typesetting Limited
Printed and bound in Great Britain by Dotesios Printers Limited,
Bradford-on-Avon, Wiltshire

Contents

Introduction	vii

PART 1 *INDEX MEDICUS* AND THE MEDLARS SERVICE

Background — 3
History of the service — 3
Coverage — 4
Journal priorities — 5
Article indexing — 5
Vocabulary — 5

Tools used in searching Index Medicus — 7
Public MeSH — 7
Annotated MeSH — 11
Tree Structures — 11
Permuted MeSH — 13
MeSH Supplementary Chemical Records (SCR) — 16

Details of headings used in MeSH — 19
Headings used in *Index Medicus* — 19
The vocabulary of MeSH — 19
   Main headings — 20
   Geographic headings — 20
   Check tags — 20
   Citation types — 20
   Non-MeSH — 20
   Minor descriptors — 21
   Entry terms — 21
   Data form abbreviations — entry versions — 21
Subheadings — 24

Difficulties in tracing the correct heading	25
Word forms	25
Anglo-American spelling	27
Term inversion	28
Alphabetisation	28
Pre-coordinated headings	28
Synonyms	29
Index Medicus	31
The monthly *Index Medicus*	33

PART 2 *EXCERPTA MEDICA*

Background	37
History	37
Coverage	37
Journal coverage	38
EM list of journals abstracted	38
Format	40
Guides to using *Excerpta Medica*	41
Malimet	41
Guide to the subject index terminology	42
Excerpta Medica classification system (*EM*clas)	43
The index to *Em*clas	45
The index to *Em*tags	45
Class A and B terms	47
Problems with the *Guide*	47
Spelling	47
Specificity of terms	47
Word forms	48
American terminology	48
Term inversion	48
The individual sections	48
The author index	49
The abstract	49
Cumulated yearly *Excerpta Medica*	50
Searching in *Excerpta Medica*	53
Conclusion	55
Subject Index	57
Index of Examples	59

Introduction

This manual is the first in a series intended to improve searching techniques in the most widely-used indexing and abstracting services in the medical sciences. No one would deny the need for indexes and abstract journals in a field which expands at the rate medicine does. *Index Medicus* and *Excerpta Medica* are two of the most widely-used sources for searching medical information. Both sift through thousands of journals and monographs and carefully arrange articles according to their subject-matter.

This manual aims to improve search techniques by highlighting possible problems and suggesting methods of overcoming them: It discusses all the aids to searching through *Index Medicus* and *Excerpta Medica*; it includes guidance in the use of Medical Subject Headings (MeSH) both Public and Annotated, Permuted MeSH and the relatively new Supplementary Chemical Records. With *Excerpta Medica*, the manual discusses the guides to the classification system, the various indices and the most effective approach to searching the hard-copy service. Searching on-line is described where necessary, but this aspect will be fully covered in a forthcoming volume in the series.

The manual is written in a down-to-earth style which aims at keeping the reader in touch with the problem in hand. It is written for students, who need to search for information for projects and dissertations; medical librarians who wish to improve their search technique, particularly those with no formal medical librarianship training; researchers in medicine; and the allied professions and practising medical personnel who need to search, and who have little time to make mistakes.

Part 1
Index Medicus and the Medlars Service

To get the most out of this guide you will need access to Public and Annotated Medical Subject Headings (MeSH), MeSH Tree Structures, Permuted MeSH, MeSH Supplementary Chemical Records and a recent copy of *Index Medicus* (cumulated and monthly). If this is not possible, sections throughout this guide will indicate what you would have found in the sources mentioned.

Background

HISTORY OF THE SERVICE

Index Medicus is, as the name suggests, an index to periodical articles in the medical sciences. Its form has changed over the years; it has been published since 1879 when it was realised that most physicians and surgeons were unable to keep up with the proliferation of medical journals. Originally, the compilation of the index was done by hand. This was a labour-intensive activity and, as the medical sciences continued to develop and expand, such service became more and more difficult, and breakdowns in the manual compilation were becoming inevitable. In the late 1950s following the successful development of the computer, the radical solution to the production problems was found.

The computer was thus employed to compile and sort the references and eventually to print the sorted citations. The references were put on tapes which, it was later realised, were available for bibliographic searching. The system developed for searching the computer tapes was called Medlars (*Med*ical *l*iterature *a*nalysis and *r*etrieval *s*ystem), and became fully operational in 1963.

Medlars is thus a biproduct of the printed or 'hard copy' version of the references. From it, three major indexes are produced: *Index Medicus*, *Index to Dental Literature* and *International Nursing Index*. In addition Medlars can produce recurring bibliographies in specialised subject areas of medicine, and retrospective searches in response to specific requests; these are called demand searches.

In 1966 the Medlars service was initiated in the UK, with off-line batch-processing being the only method of searching. In the early 1970s experimental work began on a system so that the tapes could be searched from remote terminals on-line. This led to Medline, Medlars on-line, which became available in the USA for general use in 1973 and in the UK on an experimental basis in 1974 and commercially in the same year. The searches in the UK were carried out at the Science Reference Library, Bayswater, London. Individuals booked a time and were linked directly to Elhill, USA. This was quite a stimulating time knowing that the telephone account was quickly mounting while the correct keyword was identified and typed in.

Developments since then have been rapid. BLAISE (the *British Library Automated Information SErvice*) began in 1977, and took over the running of the Medline searches for the UK.

It was soon realised that such a collection of references, accessible at remote terminals, was a commercially-interesting proposition. The National Library of Medicine, who produce the references for Medline, were approached by a number of companies with a view to mounting the Medlars tapes onto 'host' computers for access. Lockheed Dialog was the first to mount the Medline tapes, and remains a frequently used host. Data Star, a Swiss host, has also done this and there are often decisions to be made as to which host should be used.

COVERAGE

Three thousand journals are selected for indexing from the 20,000 or so received by the National Library of Medicine. This gives rise to over a quarter of a million citations each year, of which 70% are in English. About 2,500 journals are indexed for *Index Medicus*, with the remainder used to produce the *Index to Dental Literature* and the *International Nursing Index*. Since 1976, selected monographs — mainly from conferences — have also been included. The articles are in any language from over 70 countries, and are selected as the optimum number to satisfy the majority of Medlars' users. A list of the journals covered is issued each year. Since 1975 author abstracts have been added to the tapes where publishers permit this. Over 60 per cent of Medlars records have abstracts, which are available when interrogating the tapes or carrying out an on-line search, but not in *Index Medicus*.

The decentralisation of indexing is an NLM policy. Centres are selected around the world which index their own national journals. The number of centres changes, for example, Iran no longer participates while Switzerland and Colombia have been recently added to the list. The British Library indexers index over 14,000 articles a year from some 80 British journals.

JOURNAL PRIORITIES

The depth of indexing and the number of subject headings assigned to each article depends upon the priority given to the journal in which the article appears. (Headings are discussed below; see **Medical Subject Headings**.)

Primary or rush journals have the greatest depth of indexing and include the major medical journals, such as the *New England Journal of Medicine*. Secondary journals are rather more research-oriented. They are indexed, but are not assigned so many headings. Tertiary journals are primarily practical clinical and paramedical. The articles are not indexed in depth and fewer headings are assigned. Finally, some journals are indexed selectively. Articles are considered for relevance and are then treated as primary, secondary or tertiary on the articles' merits rather than the journals'. An example of a journal which is indexed selectively is *Science*.

ARTICLE INDEXING

The specialist indexers who assign headings to each article are not medically qualified unlike the indexers for *Excerpta Medica*. Less important articles, or articles from tertiary journals, get fewer subject headings: since 1981 the average number of headings has dropped to between eight and ten. Up to three headings are assigned for *Index Medicus*, these are the most important and are called print headings.

VOCABULARY

The Medlars service uses a fixed vocabulary which needs careful consideration. The vocabulary is used in *Index Medicus* to group articles together and to aid retrieval in the on-line service. Before looking at the tools used in searching we shall consider this fixed vocabulary, looking at its strengths and weaknesses.

Many databases use a free-text searching facility only. This permits the searcher to formulate his or her search in general terms but causes problems when all possible synonyms have to be searched.

Looking at an example in medicine it is easy to find diseases which have different names or are written in different forms; another area is drug names where generic, trade or chemical names may all be used in different papers to refer to the same drug.

In a fixed-text vocabulary, the guide to the correct term is called the thesaurus. It lists the preferred terms, and guides the searcher away from the non-preferred terms. Thus, if the searcher looks at the correct form of the word — say, the generic name of a drug — as specified by the thesaurus, all references in which synonyms have been used will be found together under this preferred term.

In Medlars the thesaurus is called Medical Subject Headings (MeSH).

Tools used in searching *Index Medicus*

Each of the tools is considered separately. Questions asked can be easily answered using the appropriate tool. If you are unable to obtain a specific tool, then use the examples shown in the figures which accompany the text.

MeSH contains some 16,000 main headings, cross-references, tree numbers and publication notes, and has two components: Public MeSH and Annotated MeSH.

PUBLIC MeSH

We shall consider Public MeSH first by looking at Part 2 of the January edition of *Index Medicus*. You will notice that, considering it covers the whole field of medicine, it is quite a slim volume. A compromise has been made between specificity and size, so some topics which you may wish to look up will be indexed under a more general heading than might have been anticipated. It should be noted that articles are always indexed under the most specific term available and so access to **Tree Structures** (see below) is very useful.

Look first at **Phenothiazine Tranquilizers** in Public MeSH (1984) (see Figure 1). The first thing you notice is a code number.

PHENOTHIAZINE TRANQUILIZERS
D15.236.872.331.628+
73
XU PERAZINE
XU PIPERACETAZINE
XU PIPOTHIAZINE
XU PIPOTHIAZINE PALMITATE

Figure 1. From Public MeSH

This code, D15.236.872.331.628, is followed by a +. This indicates that there are more specific items mentioned in MeSH and to identify them we need to use the Tree Structures. Under the code is the number 73. This indicates the year the term was introduced into *Index Medicus*. Following this are four XU terms. For an explanation, each of these words should now be looked up (see Figure 2). You will see that the four words *Perazine*, *Piperacetazine*, *Pipothiazine* and *Pipothiazine Palmitate* all have 'see under **Phenothiazine Tranquilizers**' as references. You may also notice that the four terms are printed

PERACETIC ACID see under ACETIC ACIDS
X ACETYL HYDROPEROXIDE
X PEROXYACETIC ACID

PERAZINE see under PHENOTHIAZINE TRANQUILIZERS

PERCEPTION
F2.463.593+
see related
SENSATION
XR SENSATION

PIPEMIDIC ACID see under NICOTINIC ACIDS
X PIPERAMIC ACID

PIPERACETAZINE see under PHENOTHIAZINE TRANQUILIZERS

PIPERACILLIN
D20.85.639.65.600
84

PIPOBROMAN
D3.383.606.773   D22.204.678
73

PIPOTHIAZINE see under PHENOTHIAZINE TRANQUILIZERS

PIPOTHIAZINE PALMITATE see under PHENOTHIAZINE TRANQUILIZERS

PIPRADOL see PIPRADROL

PIPRADROL
D3.383.621.820   D15.236.122.787
X PIPRADOL

Figure 2. From Public MeSH

in a smaller typeface. These terms are known as minor descriptors and are discussed below. At this stage it can be noted that minor descriptors will not appear as main or print headings in *Index Medicus* though they are available for searching on-line. The XU term first noted is a 'backward see under'.

Return now to **Phenothiazine Tranquilizers**. Look up this term in Annotated MeSH (see Figure 3). The tool is used for on-line searching and gives more information. There are check tags, minor descriptors, citation types and geographic headings, the history of the heading and on-line notes. Looking at the **Phenothiazine Tranquilizers**, the additional information given follows the tree code. The terms 'do not use . . .' refers to the use of subheadings. These subheadings break up the text in *Index Medicus*, but are more important as search aids in on-line searching and their use is explained below.

Now look up the four XU terms in Annotated MeSH in the same way. Here the headings are all in bold print. This shows that Annotated MeSH is for on-line searching where minor descriptors are acceptable search terms and can be treated in the same way as main headings.

Now let us take a more complicated example. Look up the term **Gamma Globulins** in Public MeSH and Annotated MeSH, and note the differences (see Figures 4.1 and 4.2).

In Public MeSH certain data are given. First, two tree codes which, as will be shown, indicate different emphases of the term. An historical note shows when the term was introduced and what it was prior to this. In the case of **Gamma Globulins**, the term was introduced in 1975; previously (1963–74) it was **Gamma Globulin** (i.e. without the final s).

When reading the annotations, it is important to note that the semicolon is the place to pause. The information between semicolons is complete in itself. The '/deficiency was **Gamma Globulin Deficiency** see under **Agammaglobulinemia** 1963–67;' is one such piece of information and informs the reader that between 1963 and 1967 there was an entry in MeSH under **Gamma Globulin Deficiency** referring the searcher to **Agammaglobulinemia**. It also informs the searcher that **Gamma Globulins** with the subheading deficiency, represented by the '/deficiency', is covered by **Agammaglobulinemia.** The notes go on to inform the searcher that **Immune Serum Globulin** was used as a heading in 1965.

PHENOTHIAZINE TRANQUILIZERS
D15.236.872.331.628 +
do not use /analogs /biosyn /defic /physiol
73
XU PERAZINE
XU PIPERACETAZINE
XU PIPOTHIAZINE
XU PIPOTHIAZINE PALMITATE

Figure 3. From Annotated MeSH

GAMMA GLOBULINS
D12.776.124.790.522   D12.776.377.715.440
75; was GAMMA GLOBULIN 1963–74; /deficiency was GAMMA GLOBULIN DEFICIENCY see under AGAMMAGLOBULINEMIA 1963–67; IMMUNE SERUM GLOBULIN was heading 1965

Figure 4.1 From Public MeSH

GAMMA GLOBULINS
D12.776.124.790.522   D12.776.377.715.440
do not use /antag /blood; /defic = AGAMMAGLOBULINEMIA or DYSGAMMAGLOBULINEMIA (TN 225); do not use /ther use; index under IMMUNIZATION, PASSIVE for ther with gamma globulins in general or unspecified; anti-gamma globulin antibodies = ANTI-ANTIBODIES (IM) + GAMMA GLOBULINS (IM): TN 224: relation to IMMUNOGLOBULINS; gammopathies or gammapathies (excessive immunoglobulins in blood) = HYPERGAMMAGLOBULINEMIA: see note there & TN 226; various gamma globulins: TN 224

75; was GAMMA GLOBULIN 1963–74; /deficiency was GAMMA GLOBULIN DEFICIENCY see under AGAMMAGLOBULINEMIA 1963–67; IMMUNE SERUM GLOBULIN was heading 1965

use GAMMA GLOBULINS to search GAMMA GLOBULIN back thru 1966; search GAMMA GLOBULIN DEFICIENCY under AGAMMAGLOBULINEMIA 1966–77

Figure 4.2 From Annotated MeSH

DENTAL SERVICE, HOSPITAL
N2.278.354.422.298   N2.421.240.200
N4.452.442.422.298
only /econ /legis /man /organ /stand /trends /util
78; was HOSPITAL DENTAL SERVICE 1963–77
use DENTAL SERVICE, HOSPITAL to search HOSPITAL DENTAL SERVICE back thru 1966
see related
    DENTAL FACILITIES
X   HOSPITAL DENTAL SERVICE

Figure 5. From Annotated MeSH

ANNOTATED MeSH

Look at the same term in Annotated MeSH. More information is given here of particular interest to the on-line searcher. Certain subheadings are not permitted and a possible problem for the indexer is spelled out by reference to a technical note TN225. Other specific instances are covered; in particular, an indication as to how to proceed with a search for antigamma globulin antibodies where the searcher is recommended to combine the two *Index Medicus (IM)* terms **Anti-Antibodies** with **Gamma Globulins.**

The remainder of that section follows the same discussion as previously given.

The next interesting section begins **Use Gamma Globulins** to search **Gamma Globulin** back through 1966. This means that for on-line searchers the change of indexing from **Gamma Globulin** to **Gamma Globulins** has been accommodated within the system. However, it should be noted that, if searching in *Index Medicus*, the old heading must be used prior to the introduction of the new heading. In this instance, the change is minimal and does not result in a significant positional change in the index.

Consider **Dental Service Hospital** for a moment, though (see Figure 5). This term was introduced in 1978. Prior to that it was **Hospital Dental Service**. Although in Annotated MeSH we can see that on-line searching requires the use of only the new term, manual searching through issues of *Index Medicus* prior to 1978 requires a radical change. Thus the two sources are necessary for selection of terms prior to searching.

We move now to the Tree Structures which help in the selection of the most specific term available.

TREE STRUCTURES

These exist separately or as the final section of Public MeSH. The 16,000 terms in MeSH appear in the Tree Structures in a polyhierarchical order. Terms are assigned to one or more broad subject headings, and are then placed in sequence. The sequence forms a semantically-related tree. If a term has more than one meaning or emphasis, it may appear in more than one position in the Tree Structures.

Any example serves to demonstrate the usefulness of the Tree Structures. However, as terms change and new terms may be added, for consistency I shall state the date of publication of the MeSH Tree Structures and MeSH Headings.

CARDIAC GLYCOSIDES
D9.203.408.180+   D18.222.175+
X   CARDIOTONIC STEROIDS
XU CONVALLARIA GLYCOSIDES

From Public MeSH

D9 — CHEMICALS AND DRUGS—CARBOHYDRATES AND HYPOGLYCEMIC AGENTS

CARBOHYDRATES AND HYPOGLYCEMIC AGENTS (NON MESH)

CARBOHYDRATES AND HYPOGLYCEMIC AGENTS (NON MESH)	D9			
CARBOHYDRATES	D9.203			
AMINO SUGARS	D9.203.67			
HEXOSAMINES	D9.203.67.342			
GALACTOSAMINE	D9.203.67.342.356			
ACETYLGALACTOSAMINE *	D9.203.67.342.356.50			
GLUCOSAMINE	D9.203.67.342.531			
ACETYLCLUCOSAMINE *	D9.203.67.342.531.50			
TUNICAMYCIN *	D9.203.67.342.531.900	D20.85.891	D20.388.913	
MEGLUMINE *	D9.203.67.342.600	D2.33.800.	D9.203.853.	
DIATRIZOATE MEGLUMINE *	D9.203.67.342.600.500	D2.33.800. D26.298.240.	D2.241.223.	D9.203.853.
IOTHALAMATE MEGLUMINE	D9.203.67.342.600.600	D2.33.800. D26.298.566.	D2.241.223.	D9.203.853.
MURAMIC ACIDS *	D9.203.67.550	D2.241.81.	D2.241.511.	D9.203.811.
ACETYLMURAMYL-ALANYL-ISOGLUTAMI	D9.203.67.550.50	D9.203.811.	D12.644.233.	D24.611.59.
NEURAMINIC ACIDS	D9.203.67.687	D2.241.81.	D2.241.511.	D9.203.811.
SIALIC ACIDS	D9.203.67.687.668	D9.203.811.	D2.241.81.	D2.241.511.
CYTIDINE MONOPHOSPHATE N-ACETYLNEURAMINIC ACID *	D9.203.67.687.668.250	D2.241.81. D13.695.740.	D2.241.511. D13.695.827.	D9.203.811.
BLOOD GLUCOSE	D9.203.147			
DEOXY SUGARS	D9.203.254			
DEOXYGLUCOSE *	D9.203.254.229			
DEOXYRIBOSE	D9.203.254.330			
FUCOSE	D9.203.254.488	D9.203.546.		
RHAMNOSE	D9.203.254.799	D9.203.546.		
DIETARY CARBOHYDRATES	D9.203.301			
GLYCOSIDES	D9.203.408			
RUTIN	D9.203.408.134.779	D11.786.170.		
HYDROXYETHYLRUTOSIDE *	D9.203.408.134.779.400			
CARDIAC GLYCOSIDES	D9.203.408.180	D18.222.175		
CANNOGENIN THEVETOSIDE *	D9.203.408.180.135	D4.808.155.	D18.222.175.	
CONVALLARIA GLYCOSIDES *	D9.203.408.180.173	D18.222.175.		
DIGITALIS GLYCOSIDES	D9.203.408.180.261	D18.222.175.		
DIGITONIN	D9.203.408.180.261.236.	D26.550.226		
DIGITOXIN	D9.203.408.180.261.336	D4.808.155.	D18.222.175.	
ACETYLDIGITOXINS *	D9.203.408.180.261.336.259	D4.808.155.	D18.222.175.	
DIGOXIN	D9.203.408.180.261.436	D4.808.155.	D18.222.175.	
ACETYLDIGOXINS *	D9.203.408.180.261.436.50	D4.808.155.	D18.222.175.	
MEDIGOXIN *	D9.203.408.180.261.436.500	D4.808.155.	D18.222.175.	
LANATOSIDES	D9.203.408.180.261.657	D18.222.175.		
DESLANOSIDE *	D9.203.408.180.261.657.200	D18.222.175.		
PROSCILLARIDIN *	D9.203.408.180.660	D4.808.122.	D18.222.175.	
STROPHANTHINS	D9.203.408.180.810	D4.808.155.	D18.222.175.	
CYMARINE *	D9.203.408.180.810.250	D4.808.155.	D18.222.175.	
OUABAIN	D9.203.408.180.810.600	D4.808.155.	D18.222.175.	
GALACTOSIDES *	D9.203.408.320			

Figure 6. Tree Structures

Consider the term **Cardiac Glycosides** (see Figure 6). Look this up in Public MeSH and Annotated MeSH and two codes are noted: D9.203.408.180+ and D18.222.175+. (The + indicates that there are more specific terms under this heading which can be found by using the Tree Codes.)

Look up both the Tree Structures for 1984 starting with D9.203.408.180. The D9 section is concerned with *Carbohydrates* and *Hypoglycaemic Agents*, a non-MeSH term which is explained below. D9.203 represents *Carbohydrates*. This term — not surprisingly — has a number of more specific terms indented beneath it. D9.203.408 is the code for *Glycosides*. Finally D9.203.408.180 represents *Cardiac Glycosides*. At this point we can see how the hierarchy is built up. Beneath *Cardiac Glycosides* we can see three terms on the same hierarchical level **Cannogenin Thevetoside**, **Convallaria Glycosides** and **Digitalis Glycosides**. There is then a further level of hierarchy and one more level for some of the terms. An asterisk (*) beside a number of these terms. These, as the footnote explains, are minor descriptors. These can be searched on-line, but are not used as print headings in *Index Medicus*.

Now look up the second tree code D18.222.175 (see Figure 7). The D18 section is concerned with *Cardiovascular Agents*, with D18.222 representing *Cardiotonic Agents* and D18.222.175 again is *Cardiac Glycosides*. The same terms are indented as they are both cardiovascular agents *and* carbohydrates. This highlights the way the same term can appear in two separate parts of the Tree Structures where the two show a different emphasis of meaning. Other examples are where an inorganic chemical such as nitroprusside is placed in section D1, *Chemicals — Inorganic*, and in a section indicating its action as a vasodilating agent in D18. If you look this term up, you will also discover that it is placed in three other sections including D26 (*Miscellaneous Drugs and Agents*) where it is shown as being used as an indicator.

PERMUTED MeSH

This gives entry points into MeSH headings from different constructs of MeSH terms. Each term is broken down into its components. These terms are rotated in an alphabetical index.

The terms selected are not only major descriptors, as can be seen if the term **Pulmonary** is considered (see Figure 8). It does

D18 — CHEMICALS AND DRUGS—CARDIOVASCULAR AGENTS

CARDIOVASCULAR AGENTS	D18			
ANTIHYPERTENSIVE AGENTS	D18.162			
PHENOXYBENZAMINE	D18.162.712	D2.92.471.	D16.848.115.	D23.846.739
PHENTOLAMINE	D18.162.721	D3.383.374.	D16.848.115.	
PRAZOSIN *	D18.162.730	D3.438.786.		
PROPRANOLOL	D18.162.738	D2.33.329. D18.97.675	D2.92.63. D18.918.792	D16.848.215.
RAUWOLFIA ALKALOIDS	D18.162.804	D3.132.973.	D3.549.937.	D16.848.415.
RESERPINE	D18.162.804.811	D3.132.973.	D3.549.937.	D16.848.415.
DESERPIDINE *	D18.162.804.811.277	D3.132.973.	D3.549.937.	D16.848.415.
RESCINNAMINE *	D18.162.804.811.809	D3.132.973.	D3.549.937.	D16.848.415.
SYROSINGOPINE	D18.162.804.811.872	D3.132.973.	D3.549.937.	D16.848.415.
SARALASIN	D18.162.878	D12.644.456.	D24.185.798.	
TEPROTIDE *	D18.162.885	D12.644.456.		
TIMOLOL	D18.162.889	D2.33.329.	D2.92.63.	D16.848.215.
TICRYNAFEN *	D18.162.891	D2.241.511.	D3.383.903.	D19.770.224.
TODRALAZINE *	D18.162.893	D2.442.925.	D3.383.710.	
TRIMETHAPHAN	D18.162.895	D3.383.374.	D16.653.396.	
TRIMETHIDINIUM COMPOUNDS *	D18.162.918	D2.92.102.	D2.675.276.	D16.653.396.
UROTENSINS *	D18.162.943	D12.644.910	D24.185.798.	
VERATRUM ALKALOIDS	D18.162.955	D3.132.920		
PROTOVERATRINES *	D18.162.955.710	D3.132.920.	D3.549.256.	
CALCIUM CHANNEL BLOCKERS	D18.192			
BENCYCLANE *	D18.192.150	D2.455.426.	D18.918.150	
DILTIAZEM *	D18.192.282	D3.438.79.	D18.918.214	
FENDILINE *	D18.192.360	D2.92.471.	D18.97.360	D18.918.360
NIFEDIPINE	D18.192.638	D3.383.725.	D18.918.638	
PERHEXILINE	D18.192.754	D3.383.621.	D18.918.754	
PRENYLAMINE	D18.192.786	D2.92.471.	D18.918.786	
VERAPAMIL	D18.192.953	D2.92.471.	D18.97.953	D18.918.925
GALLOPAMIL *	D18.192.953.395	D2.92.471.	D18.97.953.	D18.918.925
CARDIOTONIC AGENTS	D18.222			
CARDIAC GLYCOSIDES	D18.222.175	D9.203.408.		

Figure 7. Tree Structures

PULMONARY
ABSCESS, PULMONARY see LUNG ABSCESS
ADENOMATOSIS, PULMONARY, BOVINE see PNEUMONIA, ATYPICAL INTERSTITIAL, OF CATTLE
ADENOMATOSIS, PULMONARY, OVINE see PULMONARY ADENOMATOSIS, OVINE
CIRRHOSIS, PULMONARY see PULMONARY FIBROSIS
COIN LESION, PULMONARY
ECHINOCOCCOSIS, PULMONARY
EMPHYSEMA, ACUTE BOVINE PULMONARY see PNEUMONIA, ATYPICAL INTERSTITIAL, OF CATTLE
EMPHYSEMA, PULMONARY see PULMONARY EMPHYSEMA
EOSINOPHILIA, PULMONARY see PULMONARY EOSINOPHILIA
HYDATID CYST, PULMONARY see ECHINOCOCCOSIS, PULMONARY
HYDATIDOSIS, PULMONARY see ECHINOCOCCOSIS, PULMONARY
HYPERTENSION, PULMONARY
PULMONARY ADENOMATOSIS, BOVINE see PNEUMONIA, ATYPICAL INTERSTITIAL, OF CATTLE
PULMONARY ADENOMATOSIS, OVINE
PULMONARY ALVEOLAR PROTEINOSIS
PULMONARY ALVEOLI
PULMONARY ARTERY
PULMONARY ARTERY WEDGE PRESSURE see PULMONARY WEDGE PRESSURE
PULMONARY CAPILLARY WEDGE PRESSURE see PULMONARY WEDGE PRESSURE
PULMONARY CIRCULATION
PULMONARY COIN LESION see COIN LESION, PULMONARY
PULMONARY DIFFUSING CAPACITY
PULMONARY DISEASES see LUNG DISEASES
PULMONARY EDEMA
PULMONARY EMBOLISM
PULMONARY EMPHYSEMA
PULMONARY EOSINOPHILIA
PULMONARY FIBROSIS
PULMONARY GAS EXCHANGE
PULMONARY HEART DISEASE
PULMONARY NEOPLASMS see LUNG NEOPLASMS
PULMONARY NODULE, SOLITARY see COIN LESION, PULMONARY
PULMONARY SEQUESTRATION see BRONCHOPULMONARY SEQUESTRATION
PULMONARY STENOSIS see PULMONARY VALVE STENOSIS
PULMONARY STRETCH RECEPTORS see under MECHANORECEPTORS
PULMONARY SUBVALVULAR STENOSIS see under IDIOPATHIC HYPERTROPHIC SUBVALVULAR STENOSIS
PULMONARY SURFACTANT
PULMONARY VALVE
PULMONARY VALVE INSUFFICIENCY
PULMONARY VALVE STENOSIS
PULMONARY VEINS
PULMONARY VENOUS WEDGE PRESSURE see PULMONARY WEDGE PRESSURE
PULMONARY WEDGE PRESSURE
SURFACTANT, PULMONARY see PULMONARY SURFACTANT
TUBERCULOSIS, PULMONARY
VENTILATORS, PULMONARY see RESPIRATORS

Figure 8. From Permuted MeSH

not matter if the term appears at the end of a compound or the beginning — every term with **Pulmonary** as part of it, is included here. Notice **Hydatid Cyst, Pulmonary**. This is only an entry point in MeSH, not a preferred term, yet it is included in Permuted MeSH with its 'see' reference to **Echinococcosis, Pulmonary**.

Permuted MeSH is very useful if you are not sure how a term

may be arranged. For example Air Embolism (Figure 9) is not mentioned in MeSH, but under Air in Permuted MeSH, the term **Embolism, Air** is included. This shows the preferred order of the two words when searching.

AIR
   AIR
   AIR BLADDER see AIR SACS
   AIR CONDITIONING
   AIR IONIZATION
   AIR MICROBIOLOGY
   AIR MOVEMENTS
   AIR POLLUTANTS
   AIR POLLUTANTS, ENVIRONMENTAL see under AIR POLLUTANTS
   AIR POLLUTANTS, OCCUPATIONAL see under AIR POLLUTANTS
   AIR POLLUTANTS, RADIOACTIVE see under AIR POLLUTANTS
   AIR POLLUTION
   AIR POLLUTION, RADIOACTIVE
   AIR POLLUTION, TOBACCO SMOKE see TOBACCO SMOKE POLLUTION
   AIR PRESSURE see under ATMOSPHERIC PRESSURE
   AIR SACS
   AIR SWALLOWING see AEROPHAGY
   EMBOLISM, AIR
   ENVIRONMENTAL AIR POLLUTANTS see AIR POLLUTANTS, ENVIRONMENTAL
   HOSPITALS, AIR FORCE see HOSPITALS, MILITARY
   LAMINAR AIR-FLOW AREAS see ENVIRONMENT, CONTROLLED
   OCCUPATIONAL AIR POLLUTANTS see AIR POLLUTANTS, OCCUPATIONAL
   RADIOACTIVE AIR POLLUTANTS see AIR POLLUTANTS, RADIOACTIVE
   RESPIRATORS, AIR-PURIFYING see RESPIRATORY PROTECTIVE DEVICES

Figure 9. From Permuted MeSH

MeSH SUPPLEMENTARY CHEMICAL RECORDS (SCR)

This is the most recent tool introduced to help the searcher use Medlars. It became generally available in 1983 and differs from the other three tools in that it lists specific chemical names rather than broad medical subject headings. It is far more specific than MeSH and gives useful information to the searcher — for example, under what heading a particular chemical may be found in MeSH. There are some 25,000 chemicals listed, selected from articles indexed since 1970. Only chemicals which are mentioned significantly are included. The file has been searchable on-line since 1980, though articles published in the UK have only been indexed using SCR since 1981.

Entries have varying amounts of information. If you have a copy please use it. If not, information is given here which will help when a copy is available.

If we consider the term **Methylatropine**, the entry has a number of sections prefixed with a two-letter code in parentheses.

(RN) 31610-87-4   This is the *registry number* of the chemical abstracts service or the enzyme commission number (EC).

(SY) **Methyl Atropine**   There are six entries with this prefix, all are synonyms for the term. They have been identified by the indexers of the periodicals. Others can be added if and when necessary. They appear as cross-references with SCR. (Look up **Methyl Atropine** as an example.) It does not include all possible synonyms only those cited in the indexed journals.

(HM) *****Atropine Derivatives**   This is a particularly useful section. The letters HM stand for *Heading Mapped* and refers the searcher to the appropriate MeSH heading acceptable for searching in *Index Medicus*.

(PA) **Antimuscarinic Agent**   This section gives the *pharmacological* action of the cited chemical. There may be more than one (PA) section.

(NO)   Here are added notes to aid the indexing of the substance. They are also useful for the searchers unsure of, for example, registry numbers of stereo isomers. In the example chosen, several registry numbers are given.

A section not included under **Methylatropine** is the indexing instruction (II) section. This contains MeSH headings alone or in combination with subheadings which may qualify the term but are not pharmacological actions. They are terms which should be considered when indexing.

17

When chemicals, agents or drugs are given in combination in, say, cancer chemotherapy, the combination is often given an acronym to identify it. This acronym, if used in papers, will appear in the SCR. For example ROAP, which is a combination of vincristine rubidazone, cytarabine and prednisone in the treatment of leukaemia appears under ROAP with, consequently, four (HM) fields.

The named product can be searched for on-line using the code (NM) following the Name of Substance.

Details of Headings Used in MeSH

The first two sections have covered the four main tools used to exploit Medlars, namely Public MeSH, Annotated MeSH, Permuted MeSH and MeSH Supplementary Chemical Records. This section deals with the detail of the headings used in MeSH, with their definitions.

If for any reason the use of the tools mentioned is not completely clear, please reread them now.

HEADINGS USED IN *INDEX MEDICUS*

These are updated annually. New headings are added and some existing headings may be deleted or changed depending on usage. For example the heading **AIDS** was a term found in references in mid-year. This meant that though articles could be indexed for Medline almost immediately, the term was not shown in MeSH until January of the following year.

Generally, a suitable heading can be found in MeSH. If you are not sure which heading may be used check in MeSH first. Think of a broader heading and then use MeSH Tree Structures. Use Permuted MeSH if available. If a chemical is being searched use SCR and find the *Index Medicus* heading.

THE VOCABULARY OF MeSH

There are five types of major descriptor, the term given to

MeSH headings which are used to index articles for Medlars. They are the terms which can be used to retrieve articles from the service. Not all are available in *Index Medicus*, though all can be searched on-line.

MAIN HEADINGS

These are the headings which can be printed in *Index Medicus* and under which relevant articles are placed. An example of a main heading is **Gamma Globulins**.

GEOGRAPHIC HEADINGS

These are grouped under category Z of the MeSH Tree Structures. They are never printed in *Index Medicus* and are used for indexing when the location is an important aspect of the article. Geographic headings are used mainly in the field of epidemiology. For example, the geographic headings shown in section Z1 are all acceptable search terms on-line but articles are only indexed under one of these headings if the article has the geographic region as a major facet of the article. 'Prevalence of Schistosomiasis in Namibia' would use the geographic heading; whereas 'Treatment of Schistosomiasis in a Namibian Hospital' would not, unless the hospital's treatment was unique and the Namibian context was an important aspect.

CHECK TAGS

These are the routine concepts such as **Animal, Case Report, Female, Human**, etc. Again, they are never used as *Index Medicus* headings, though they are available for on-line searching where a refinement is necessary.

CITATION TYPES

These are used to indicate the form of the article or some specific aspect of it — for example, *English Abstract, Monograph, Review* — all useful when searching on-line when only reviews for example, are required.

NON-MeSH

These are indicated in the MeSH Tree Structures by the words 'non-MeSH' in parentheses. They are words placed in the Trees for structural reasons. They are not available for indexing but are useful to group the Tree Structure headings.

Look up E1.302 **Diagnosis, Respiratory System (non-MeSH)**. It is structurally necessary as a broader term to **Bronchography** down to **Respiratory Sounds**. They are added to the Medline database for convenient headings to 'explode'. Using this technique permits the searcher to access articles indexed under all the more specific terms, and it saves the searcher time in inputting all narrower terms for the search.

MINOR DESCRIPTORS

These terms are 'see under' references. They can be used for searching on-line, but not in *Index Medicus*. If the main part of an article is concerned with a heading accepted as a minor descriptor, there will be a 'see under' reference to guide the searcher to the relevant major descriptor.

If all minor descriptors were used in *Index Medicus*, the index would become unmanageable. There has to be a compromise between the number of headings and the size of the index.

ENTRY TERMS

In order to assist the searcher find the most appropriate main headings, a 'see' reference is used. This guides the searcher from a non-preferred or 'entry' term to a preferred term or main heading. The entry term is not used to store references even in the on-line service. However, searchers who use the term on-line will be automatically mapped to the appropriate main heading. It is not only a synonym guide but also guides from possible specific entry points to a more general main heading. For example, look up **Psychiatry, Military** also **Rachitis** (Figure 10).

DATA FORM ABBREVIATIONS — ENTRY VERSIONS

These are abbreviations of headings indicated by the prefix DF: in Annotated MeSH. They are mainly for the convenience of indexers, but are also available for searching. Look up **Lactate Dehydrogenase** in Annotated MeSH (Figure 11). Amongst the information supplied, is DF: LDH.

PSYCHIATRY
F4.96.544+   G2.403.642+
G2.403.790.600+
SPEC only: SPEC qualif; do not confuse with MENTAL DISORDERS
CATALOG: do not use /in adolesc (= ADOLESCENT PSYCHIATRY)
/in inf (= CHILD PSYCHIATRY)

PSYCHIATRY, BIOLOGICAL see BIOLOGICAL PSYCHIATRY
F4.96.544.90   G2.403.642.100

PSYCHIATRY, COMMUNITY see COMMUNITY PSYCHIATRY
F4.96.544.215+   G2.403.642.150+

PSYCHIATRY, GERIATRIC See GERIATRIC PSYCHIATRY
F4.96.544.380   G2.403.642.260

PSYCHIATRY, MILITARY see MILITARY PSYCHIATRY
F4.96.544.480   G2.403.642.508

PSYCHIC ENERGIZERS see ANTIDEPRESSIVE AGENTS
D15.236.122+

PSYCHICAL RESEARCH see PARAPSYCHOLOGY
F2.607+   F4.96.462

RACEMASES
D8.586.399.788
GEN only; see Tree D8 under ISOMERASES & choose the most specific;
do not use /analogs /defic /physiol
(75)
search ISOMERASES 1966–74
see under ISOMERASES

RACHITIS see RICKETS
C5.116.198.816+   C18.452.174.845+
C18.654.223.133.770.734

RACIAL STOCKS
11.76.368.763+
GEN; only /class /hist; policy: Manual 30.10-30.12
68

Figure 10. To demonstrate 'see' references using Annotated MeSH

LACTATE DEHYDROGENASE
D8.586.682.47.547+
do not use /analogs; DF: LDH
X   LACTIC CYTOCHROME REDUCTASE

Figure 11. To demonstrate acceptable abbreviations using Annotated MeSH

TOPICAL SUBHEADINGS WITH SCOPE NOTES AND ALLOWABLE CATEGORIES

abnormalities   (A1-9, A13-15)
   Used with organs for congenital defects producing changes in the morphology of the organ.

administration & dosage   (D)
   Used with drugs for dosage forms, routes of administration, frequency and duration of administration, quantity of medication, and the effects of these factors.

adverse effects   (D-E, F4, G3, H1, J)
   Used with drugs, chemicals, or biological agents in accepted dosage, — or with physical agents or manufactured products in normal usage, — when intended for diagnostic, therapeutic, prophylactic or anesthetic purposes. Used also for adverse effects or complications of diagnostic, therapeutic, prophylactic, anesthetic, surgical, or other procedures.

analogs & derivatives   (D1-7, D9-26)
   Used with drugs and chemicals for substances that share the same parent molecule or have similar electronic structure but differ by the addition or substitution of other atoms or molecules. Used when the specific chemical heading is not available, and no appropriate group heading exists.

analysis   (A, B1, B3-6, C4, D, G3, J)
   Used for the identification or quantitative determination of a substance or its constituents and metabolites; includes the chemical analysis of tissues, tumors, body fluids, organisms, plants, air, water, or other environmental carrier. Applies to both methodology and results. For analysis of substances in blood, cerebrospinal fluid, and urine the specific subheading designating the fluid is used.

anatomy & histology   (A, B1-2, B5-6)
   Used with organs, regions, and tissues for normal descriptive anatomy and histology; used for normal anatomy and structure of animals and plants.

antagonists & inhibitors   (D)
   Used with chemicals, drugs, and endogenous substances to indicate substances or agents which counteract their biological effects by any mechanism.

biosynthesis   (D)
   Used for the formation of chemical substances in organisms, in living cells, or by subcellular fractions.

blood   (B2, C-D, F3)
   Used for the presence or analysis of substances in the blood; also for examination of, or changes in, the blood in disease states. Excludes serodiagnosis, for which the subheading 'diagnosis' is used, and serology, for which 'immunology' is used.

blood supply   (A1-6, A8-10, A13-16, C4)
   Used for arterial, capillary, and venous systems of an organ or region whenever the specific heading for the vessel does not exist; includes blood flow through the organ.

cerebrospinal fluid   (B2, C-D, F3)
   Used for the presence or analysis of substances in the cerebrospinal fluid; also for examination of or changes in cerebrospinal fluid in disease states.

chemical synthesis   (D)
   Used for the chemical preparation of molecules in vitro. For the formation of chemical substances in organisms, living cells, or subcellular fractions, 'biosynthesis' is used.

*used only in cataloging

Figure 12. From Annotated MeSH to show allowable categories

There are a number of other sections which are more concerned with the work of the indexer. These can all be read in the opening pages of Annotated MeSH.

SUBHEADINGS

The section on subheadings in Annotated MeSH should be referred to. Find this using the contents under 'Topical Subheadings with Scope Notes and allowable Categories'. We shall refer to this and other related tables in this section.

There are 76 subheadings used to break up the references in *Index Medicus* or to refine searches on Medline. Not all 76 are allowed with every main heading and the topical subheadings list shows the allowable categories. The categories referred to in brackets such as '(A1-9, A13-15)' are the Tree Structure categories (see Figure 12). In this case, the subheading 'abnormalities' is permitted as a subheading and as a search term on-line for headings which are grouped in categories A1-9 and A13-15 only. No other heading can be given this subheading. This means that even though it may, on occasion, seem relevant and useful to use a particular subheading with a descriptor, if that descriptor is not in an allowable category, the subheading cannot be used to index and thus to search on-line.

There are many examples of subheadings being restricted for rational reasons. These are identified at the main descriptor position in Annotated MeSH. Look up **Paraquat** in Annotated MeSH (Figure 13). It belongs to category D3 (Chemicals— Organic, Heterocyclic Compounds). The category has restrictions generally but **Paraquat** and other similar compounds have the additional restrictions of not permitting the use of biosynthesis, deficiency and physiology, all of which would have been permitted according to the topical subheading lists. The restrictions in this case are reasonable.

PARAQUAT
D3.383.725.762.621   D5.723.366.656
do not use /biosyn /defic /physiol
73(71)
X   METHYL VIOLOGEN

Figure 13. From Annotated MeSH to show restrictions

Another reason for additional restrictions in the use of subheadings arises if an acceptable compound term already exists. For example, there is a subheading *Injuries* allowable for terms within the categories A1-9 and A13-15. The main headings **Head, Arm, Leg**, etc. all belong to the category A1, but have a restriction in the use of the subheading *Injury* as the compound terms **Head Injuries, Arm Injuries** and **Leg Injuries** all exist as main headings. Similarly a number of terms, such as **Gamma Globulins**, restrict the use of the subheading *Deficiency* as an acceptable term which exists for this condition. Certain arbitrary restrictions are noted with some main headings such as **Vaccines**. It is always better to check in Annotated MeSH before applying a subheading.

DIFFICULTIES IN TRACING THE CORRECT HEADING

WORD FORMS

Unfortunately MeSH can cause problems in finding headings as there are some apparent inconsistencies with the use of terminology. Many of these arise because of the use of terms by different authors.

MeSH uses vocabulary derived from a variety of languages. This would not be a problem except that the same word may be derived from Latin, Greek *and* Anglo-Saxon. This is best seen using kidney as an example (Figure 14). Using medical common sense, it will be seen that the terms renal, kidney and nephro can all be used in certain circumstances. For the non-medical searcher such apparent inconsistencies can at best be irritating, at worst a barrier between the searcher and the information.

Look up the term **Kidney** in Annotated MeSH. In the notes which follow, the indexer and searcher are asked to consider **Renal Circulation** rather than use the subheading '/blood supply'. Also they are asked to consider **Nephrectomy** rather than use the subheading '/Surgery'. When the term is referring directly to the organ, the Anglo-Saxon form is generally chosen.

Consider **Kidney Diseases**, a general term. However specific diseases will be found under neph or renal (e.g. **Nephritis** and **Nephrosclerosis**); but compare this with **Kidney Cortex Necrosis** and **Renal Osteodystrophy**.

The only general rule that can be given is to think of other terms and read the notes in Annotated MeSH. Other examples can be found in the same area — liver/hepatic, heart/cardiac, etc. Cross-references are available to assist the searcher.

KIDNEY
A5.810.453+

kidney tissue or cells in cultures: Manual 18.6.15, 18.7.2, 22.26.1, 26.33+; fetal or embryonic kidney tissue or cells in culture: do not use /embryol with KIDNEY; /blood supply: consider also RENAL CIRCULATION; /surg: consider NEPHRECTOMY; /transpl: do not coord with TRANSPLANTATION, HOMOLOGOUS unless particularly discussed; inflammation = NEPHRITIS; Goldblatt kidney: index under HYPERTENSION, RENAL; consider terms under REN- & NEPHR- CATALOG: form qualif = NEPHROLOGY /form

/transplantation was KIDNEY TRANSPLANTATION 1963-65
see related
    DIURESIS
    NEPHRECTOMY

KIDNEY, ARTIFICIAL
E7.858.82.585

do not use /instrum /methods /util (except by MeSH definition)
see related
    HEMODIALYSIS
    PERITONEAL DIALYSIS
XR HEMODIALYSIS
XR PERITONEAL DIALYSIS

KIDNEY BEAN LECTINS see PHYTOHEMAGGLUTININS
D12.776.765.677   D24.185.526.545.711
D24.310.545.711   D24.611.125.44.545.711

KIDNEY CALCULI
C12.777.419.373   C12.777.809.503

KIDNEY CALICES
A5.810.453.537.503
(75)
search KIDNEY PELVIS 1968-74
see under KIDNEY PELVIS

KIDNEY CIRCULATION see RENAL CIRCULATION
G9.330.163.812

KIDNEY COLLECTING DUCTS see KIDNEY TUBULES, COLLECTING
A5.810.453.736.560.510

KIDNEY CONCENTRATING ABILITY
G8.852.553
only /drug eff /rad eff
70(67)
    X   URINE CONCENTRATING ABILITY

KIDNEY CORTEX
A5.810.453.324
74(73)

KIDNEY CORTEX NECROSIS
C12.777.419.393
67; was NECROSIS, RENAL CORTICAL 1964-66 (Prov)
use KIDNEY CORTEX NECROSIS to search NECROSIS, RENAL CORTICAL back thru 1966 (as Prov 1966)
    X   RENAL CORTICAL NECROSIS

KIDNEY, CYSTIC
C4.182.394+   C12.777.419.413+
differentiate from KIDNEY, POLYCYSTIC; /anal /blood supply /secret /ultrastruct permitted

KIDNEY DISEASES
C12.777.419+
GEN; inflamm dis = NEPHRITIS; consider diseases under NEPHR- & RENAL; 'renal failure' not specified as 'acute' or 'chronic': check text for clues in notes under KIDNEY FAILURE, ACUTE & KIDNEY FAILURE, CHRONIC & if not able to determine, index as KIDNEY DISEASES; 'end-stage renal disease': index under KIDNEY FAILURE, CHRONIC CATALOG: form qualif = NEPHROLOGY /form
XR NEPHROLOGY

Figure 14. From Annotated MeSH to demonstrate language problems

ANGLO-AMERICAN SPELLING

A problem arises when English words are selected for searching, as there may be an American equivalent. In MeSH there is usually a cross-reference from the English to the American.

Look up **Cot Death** (Figure 15). This is in small print indicating an entry point not available for searching in *Index Medicus* although it will be mapped to the appropriate heading for on-line searching. In this case the main heading is **Sudden Infant Death**. Under this term are three entry points identified by 'X'. These are **Cot Death, Crib Death** and **SID**. In this example, we have been channelled to the preferred main heading.

Now look up **Nappy Rash** or **Napkin Rash**. There is no cross-reference to the preferred main heading which, as you may have guessed, is **Diaper Rash**.

COT DEATH see SUDDEN INFANT DEATH
C23.240.322.500

COTININE
D3.383.773.812.180
do not use /biosyn /defic /physiol; /analogs NIM only
(75)
see under PYRROLIDINONES

Figure 15. From Annotated MeSH to demonstrate American word forms

---

American spelling can also lead to problems to alphabetisation. For example, consider the English spelling **Oestrogen**. There is no cross-reference at this point to **Estrogen**, the American spelling, which is used. **Amebiasis** does have a cross-reference from **Amoebiasis** however, as does **Amobarbital** from **Amylobarbital**, etc.

There are also differences in American concepts, such as **Family Practice** rather than **General Practice**. A glance at Category N in the Tree Structures — for example, N2.278.354.180 **Financial Management Hospital** — indicates the differences in the health-care terminology. Again the only advice that can usefully be given is to be aware of the problem and take care.

TERM INVERSION

This is the technique for placing some compound terms in natural word order and others in inverted order. If in doubt, look up each part of the compound in Permuted MeSH. This shows the acceptable order.

As we saw above, the compound Air Embolism is not cross-referenced in MeSH to the main heading **Embolism, Air** but it does appear in Permuted MeSH under Air. Similarly with other terms such as **Background Radiaton**, where there is no cross-reference from **Radiation, Background**. With Brain Abscess, there is no cross-reference from Abscess, Brain. This may seem surprising as there is a cross-reference to Brain Abscess from Abscess, Cerebral. Other abscesses are indexed in their inverted form such as Abscess, Peritonsillar, so care is obviously needed. Again, Permuted MeSH is a useful tool to overcome inversions.

ALPHABETISATION

If you remember that prefixes are ignored when headings are placed in alphabetical order, no problems will arise. Using Annotated MeSH, 1984 **3- Mercaptopropionic Acid** is listed as though the '3-' did not exist. Similarly, **3- Aminopropionic Acid. P- Aminosalicylic Acid** appears under A not P.

When a letter or number appears in the body of the main heading, again the alphabetisation ignores it. For example, **Protein O-Methyltransferase** appears *after* **Protein Methyltransferase III** and *before* **Protein Methyltransferases.**

PRE-COORDINATED HEADINGS

Indexers use pre-coordinated headings wherever available. It should be noted that many three- and four-word coordinations exist. For example, **Forms and Records Control, Growth and Embryonic Development (non-MeSH)**. Other compound headings which may not have been considered are **Tuberculosis in Childhood** and **Prenatal Exposure, Delayed Effects**. For the latter using Permuted MeSH, the precoordinated term will be discovered under **Prenatal, Exposure, Delayed** or **Effects**.

SYNONYMS

Many synonyms will be used as entry points to guide the user to the main heading. However, many more which may be frequently used, are not. Some are obscured. This happens when no specific entry point is given but the synonym is found in annotations. In Public or Annotated MeSH, for example, there is no entry for the EMI scanner. A little searching, however, will show that the EMI scanner is used for tomography. Under **Tomography, X-Ray Computed** in Public MeSH there is no reference of any kind to EMI. However, in Annotated MeSH, among the annotations is a reference to CAT, EMI, ACTA and DELTA scanners which are all indexed here. This could naturally cause problems and care should be taken by finding the most acceptable broad heading and then checking the annotations.

Generally, the tools should be used together to trace the correct headings. Use the Tree Structures to find more specific terms, or broader headings. Permuted MeSH has a useful place for finding the correct form of a term particularly when terms are compound. Annotated MeSH is principally used for on-line searching but the additional information given in the annotations are often useful for the searcher of the hard copy.

Index Medicus

The first three sections have explained the strengths and weaknesses of the tools used for searching *Index Medicus* and Medline. The hard copy itself has one or two interesting points which should be noted.

First, the years' cumulated *Index Medicus*. It would be very useful if you could look at these. These are published as a single volume divided into a number of parts. In the cumulated *Index Medicus*, 1983 vol. (24) there are 14 parts.

Part 1 comprises the MeSH headings followed by the Tree Structures. Part 2 is subdivided into three sections: (1) a list of the journals and monographs indexed; (2) a Bibliography of Medical Reviews; and (3) the first part of the Author Section.

Before reading further, look at this part of the cumulated *Index Medicus*.

The List of Journals and Monographs Indexed first gives the abbreviations used, in alphabetical order. Details of the correct title are also given here at the abbreviated heading's position. Journals which are indexed selectively only are indicated by an 's'. Following the list of abbreviated titles is a full-title listing, again in alphabetical order. This gives the abbreviated heading at the full-title position. The list of abbreviated headings is particularly useful as *Index Medicus* uses these abbreviations in all citations.

If you look up *JAMA* in the abbreviations, you will appreciate the slight difficulty which may be encountered in the alphabetisation; you will also see that its full title is *Journal of the American Medical Association*. Looking this up in the full listing you find that the accepted full title is *JAMA. Journal of the American Medical Association (Chicago)*. (The 'The' of the title is ignored.)

Articles which are well-documented surveys of the recent biomedical literature are included in the Bibliography of Medical Reviews (the second section of Part 2). Reviews are arranged under MeSH headings with the same subheading as previously described. Certain 'special case' reviews, e.g. epidemiological surveys, are excluded. The exclusions are listed in the introduction to the section.

The same 'see' and 'see under' references are included.

The advantage of keeping the reviews separate is obvious. In research a review is often the best starting point, so looking up **Bibliography** will provide a list of bibliographies in various subjects.

Look up **Furans** in the Medical Reviews section (see Figure 16). You will see that there is a general review first with full citation, followed by the number of references. (If you wish to know the meaning of the abbreviated title *Clin Pharm*, check in the Abbreviations.) The first subheading used in this example is **Pharmacodynamics** where two reviews are listed. The second review is enclosed in square brackets which indicates that it is written in a language other than English. The second subheading is **Therapeutic Use**, where again there are two reviews listed, the second one being in German. All give the number of references.

FURANS
Ranitidine: a new H2-receptor antagonist. Berner BD, et al. **Clin Pharm** 1982 Nov–Dec; 1(6):499–509 (102 ref.)

PHARMACODYNAMICS
Perturbation of vesicular traffic with the carboxylic ionophore monensin. Tartakoff AM. Cell 1983 Apr; 32(4):1026–8 (14 ref.)
[New generation of histamine H2 receptor blockaders] Radbil' OS, et al. **Sov Med** 1982;(12):80–5 (58 ref.)
(Rus)

THERAPEUTIC USE
Ranitidine: a review of its pharmacology and therapeutic use in peptic ulcer disease and other allied diseases. Brogden RN, et al. **Drugs** 1982 Oct;24(4):267–303 (198 ref.)
[New ulcer drugs: is cimetidine out of date?] Fimmel CJ, et al. **Ther Umsch** 1982 Nov;39(11):841–51 (68 ref.) (Eng. Abstr.) (Ger)

Figure 16. From the bibliography of medical reviews Cumulated *Index Medicus*

Within the citation there is only one author given, followed by the words *et al*. As the cited author may not be the head of the team or the most important worker, it is usually important to find the co-authors. This brings us to the author listing. In this and each of the following four parts of volume 24 (1983), the full list of authors is given in alphabetical order.

If we try to find the co-authors of the review article under the MeSH heading **Furans** entitled 'Ranitidine: a new H_2-receptor antagonist' by Berner B. D. *et al*. First, look up **Berner B. D.** in the appropriate part or book of volume 24 (Book 2) (Figure 17). You will see that there are three co-authors. The full bibliographic citation is included here, which enables a precise check.

Berner BD, Conner CS, Sawyer DR, Siepler JK: Ranitidine: a new H2-receptor antagonist. Clin Pharm 1982 Nov-Dec; 1(6):499–509 (102 ref.)

Figure 17. From the author index of Cumulated *Index Medicus*

Books 7 to 14 of the cumulated *Index Medicus* arrange the year's citation in alphabetical order of subject heading. Looking again at **Furans** in volume 24, we find we require Book 10. Look up this term, and the whole of 1983's *Index Medicus* articles are collected here, including the reviews mentioned above. As with the reviews, all non-English-language articles are indicated by square brackets. If an English abstract is given, this is shown as **Eng. Abstr.** in parentheses. The language of the article is shown in bold type at the end of the citation. For an example of this, see **Furans**, vol.24, Book 10 [Friedel — Crafts reactions of furones and furandiones].

THE MONTHLY *INDEX MEDICUS*

Index Medicus is published monthly and each issue contains information which becomes available in the cumulated volume. MeSH is distributed with the January Part 2 of *Index Medicus*. This first part has the list of journals indexed as a separate section. The introduction in each monthly issue gives information available in Book 1 of the Cumulated *Index Medicus*, including a list of the non-English-language abbreviations used for citations. The first major section of each monthly part is the bibliography of medical reviews. The same

FURANS

Application of MDPF and fluorescamine XV chiroptical properties of MDPF condensation compounds with dipeptides in situ. Toome V, et al. **Biochem Biophys Res Commun** 1983 Jul 29;114(2):433–9

Ranitidine: a new H2-receptor antagonist. Berner BD, et al. **Clin Pharm** 1982 Nov–Dec;1(6):499–509 (102 ref.)

Diffusion of phenol in the presence of a complexing agent, tetrahydrofuran. Dressman JB, et al. **J Pharm Sci** 1983 Jan; 72(1):12–7

Ranitidine (ZANTAC). **Med Lett Drugs Ther** 1982 Dec 24; 24(625):111–3

[Friedel-Crafts reactions of furanones and furandiones] Canevet JC, et al. **Ann Pharm Fr** 1983 Feb;40(5):481–7 (Eng. Abstr.) **(Fre)**

[Formation of local changes in concentrations of hydrogen and potassium ions in bilayer lipid membranes adjacent to the membrane in the presence of monensin and nigericin] Antonenko IuN, et al. **Biofizika** 1983 Jan–Feb;28(1):56–60 (Eng. Abstr.) **(Rus)**

ADMINISTRATION & DOSAGE

H2 receptor antagonists — cimetidine and ranitidine [letter] **Br Med J [Clin Res]** 1983 Apr 16;286(6373):1283

Ranitidine in the treatment of duodenal and prepyloric ulcer: comparison of two dosage regimens. Brunner H, et al. **J Int Med Res** 1983;11(3):167–72

Influence of gamma-butyrolactone on behavior due to dopaminergic drugs. Dougherty GG, et al. **Physiol Behav** 1983 Apr;30(4):607–9

[Comparative efficacy of ranitidine and cimetidine in the short-term treatment of duodenal ulcer (results of an international controlled trial)] Laverdant C. **Gastroenterol Clin Biol** 1983 May;7(5):480–6 (Eng. Abstr.) **(Fre)**

[Functional results of oral dusodril therapy of obliterating arteriopathy of the lower extremities. Comparison of the angiogram, plethysmogram and Doppler ultrasound] Weidinger P. **Med Welt** 1983 Apr 29;34(17):531–4 **(Ger)**

[Effect of 4-week oral administration of ranitidine, a new histamine H2-receptor antagonist, on pancreatic exocrine secretion in rats] Tada H, et al. **Nippon Shokakibyo Gakkai Zasshi** 1983 Jan;80(1):98–104 (Eng. Abstr.) **(Jpn)**

ADVERSE EFFECTS

Cardiovascular toxicity of ionophores used as feed additives. Pressman BC, et al. **Adv Exp Med Biol** 1983;161:543–61

H2 receptor antagonists–cimetidine and ranitidine [letter] Rowley-Jones D, et al. **Br Med J [Clin Res]** 1983 Mar 26;286(6370):1059

Adverse effects of ranitidine therapy [letter] Cleator IG. **Can Med Assoc J** 1983 Sep 1;129(5):405

Gynecomastia and bradycardia: side effects of ranitidine? [letter] Schifman C. **Clin Pharm** 1983 May–Jun;2(3):209

The sensitizing capacity of Alstroemeria cultivars in man and guinea pig. Remarks on the occurrence, quantity and irritant and sensitizing potency of their constituents tuliposide A and tulipalin A (alpha-methylene-gamma-butyrolactone). Hausen BM, et al. **Contact Dermatitis** 1983 Jan;9(1):46–54

Ranitidine and side effects. Jawad F. **JPMA** 1983 Apr;33(4):79–80

Histamine H2 antagonists and the heart [letter] Jack D, et al. **Lancet** 1982 Dec 4;2(8310):1281–2

What ever happened to Glaxo's shares? Kilgour A. **Lancet** 1982 Oct 16;2(8303):868–9

More about ranitidine and hyperprolactinaemia [letter] Lombardo L. **Lancet** 1983 Jul 2;2(8340):42–3

Ranitidine side-effects [letter] Moebius UM. **Lancet** 1982 Nov 6;2(8306):1053–4

Symptomatic bradycardia in association with H2-receptor antagonists [letter] Shah RR. **Lancet** 1982 Nov 13;2(8307):1108

Figure 18. From Cumulated *Index Medicus*

MeSH headings and subheadings, are used throughout. Following this section is the *Index Medicus* Subject Section corresponding to the Subject Indexes of the cumulated volume. The final section of each monthly part is the *Index Medicus* Author Section, which again lists the authors of a particular article in full.

Part 2
Excerpta Medica

To get the most out of this guide to the use of *Excerpta Medica,* you will need access to the *Excerpta Medica (EM) List of Journals Abstracted, EM Guide to the Classification and Indexing System,* an annual cumulated index issue of *EM* and one of the individual parts. Examples will be given to explain points raised.

Background

HISTORY

Excerpta Medica was founded in 1946. The pioneers were physicians who wished to further the progress of medical knowledge by disseminating medical information in English. The employment of physicians to bring the medical information to the user is one of the unique features of *EM*.

As with *Index Medicus*, the compilation of the hard copy is carried out after compilation of the database; this is called Embase. All editorial work is carried out in Amsterdam for the Elsevier Science Publishers of which *EM* is a part. Embase is used to produce sources for both current awareness, in the form of core journals and the drug information service bulletins, and retrospective literature searches in the form of the abstract journals and literature indexes. Embase can be interrogated directly via a number of host systems including Data-Star, BRS, Dialog and DIMDI with a selective search availability on ESA-IRS. Different hosts may organise the files differently for on-line searching including different time-periods within files.

COVERAGE

Excerpta Medica covers all aspects of human medicine, including aspects of chemistry, sociology, management and economics where these impinge on medicine. Areas such as the environment and pollution control are also covered when relevant. Therefore, although nursing and veterinary sciences are excluded, the basic medical sciences are supplemented by developmental sciences and sociology. Within the basic sciences, two areas which have become priorities are drugs and toxicology. The term drug is taken in its widest sense to cover pharmaceuticals and other chemicals affecting humans. Toxicology covers all aspects of clinical and experimental medicine. Food additives are also included.

JOURNAL COVERAGE

About 3,500 biomedical journals are screened from cover to cover by assignment editors in Amsterdam. Other institutions scan between 15,000 and 20,000 titles for information relevant to the environment and toxicology. From this second large collection some 3,000 additional articles are added to the database annually.

Over 95 per cent of the database is compiled from journal articles, with the remainder coming from annuals, books, dissertations and monographs. There is no coverage of patent literature, which may seem surprising when first indications of new prosthetic devices appear in this form of literature.

EM LIST OF JOURNALS ABSTRACTED

This is available in hard copy, microfiche and on magnetic tape. If you have a copy of the 1984 edition, please use it here.

The list has an introduction, a statistical breakdown of the contribution of journals per country of origin, a list of new titles added since the previous edition, and the full journal list. The list includes all journals which are currently taken and screened by *Excerpta Medica*, and all those titles which have been used to compile the database.

Looking for a specific journal can be a problem, as the alphabetisation is by abbreviated title; for example, the *Journal of the American Medical Association* is not listed under its full title or *JAMA* as with *Index Medicus*, but is found under *J. Am. Med. Assoc.* Punctuation can lead to missed titles as punctuation marks are sorted before letters so the *New England Journal of Medicine* comes before *Nature* as the former is abbreviated to *N. Engl. J. Med.*, and *N.* comes at the beginning of the 'N' section.

>
> J. AM. COLL. NUTR. - JONUD* - New York USA
> Journal of the American College of Nutrition
> + J. AM. CONCRETE INST. - JACIA - Detroit USA
> Journal of the American Concrete Institute
> ● J. AM. DIET. ASSOC. - JADAA** Chicago USA
> Journal of the American Dietetic Association
> ● J. AM. GERIATR. SOC. - JAGSA** - New York USA
> Journal of the American Geriatrics Society
> ● J. AM. MED. ASSOC. - JAMAA** - Chicago USA
> Journal of the American Medical Association

Figure 19. From the list of journals abstracted by *Excerpta Medica*

The five-letter code which follows the abbreviation is the international coden. The *J. Am. Med. Assoc's* coden is *JAMAA*. This coden can be searched on-line and remains the same even if the journal title changes. (See Figure 19).

Looking again at this example, the data given per entry are:

1. the abbreviated title,
2. the five-letter coden,
3. the city and country of publication,
4. the full title.

The asterisks following the coden of *JAMAA* refer to *Excerpta Medica*'s screening policy. As there are two it means that all original articles and significant contributions are normally included in the database. A journal such as *Indian Med. Gaz.* (*The Indian Medical Gazette*) has one asterisk following the coden *IMGAA* (see Figure 20). This indicates that only certain

>
> INDIAN MED. GAZ. - IMGAA* - Calcutta India
> Indian Medical Gazette
>
> +PLAST. ENG. - PLEGB - Stamford USA
> Plastics Engineering
>
> +J. AM. OIL CHEM. SOC. - JAOCA - Chicago USA
> Journal of the American Oil Chemists' Society

Figure 20. From the list of journals abstracted for *Excerpta Medica*

articles are taken; in other words, the journal is screened selectively. Absence of an asterisk, as in the case of *Plast. Eng.* (*Plastics Engineering*) means that the journal is being evaluated. Two other codes which appear in the list are a '+' and a '•'. The + designates journals which are screened for *Excerpta Medica* in libraries in the Netherlands. These are primarily for the environment and toxicology. The • indicates journals of special importance selected by *Excerpta Medica* for rapid input of citations and abstracts. An example of this is *J. Am. Med. Assoc.* The + can be seen with *J. Am. Oil Chem. Soc.*

A further listing which also covers books and is arranged in full title order is available on microfiche.

FORMAT

Whereas the printed version of Medlars *Index Medicus* is published as a monthly index, the printed version of *Excerpta Medica* is published as 44 abstract journals and two drug-related literature indexes. These provide coverage of human medicine and aspects of basic biological science. Each abstract journal covers one area (e.g. cancer) and is called a section. The sections are built up from a number of issues per year into a volume. A single article entered in the *EM* system can be indexed in more than one section if there is more than one aspect to the article. This will be discussed again when considering the on-line Embase in a future volume.

Guides to using *Excerpta Medica*

The most useful aid to searching *Excerpta Medica* is the *Guide to the Classification and Indexing System*. A new format was introduced in 1983 using coloured pages to identify the different sections. There are two indices — an alphabetical index of all of the concepts contained in the classification system and an alphabetical listing of the most frequently used terms in the subject indices of each of the abstract journals which make up *Excerpta Medica*. Many of the entry points within this latter listing are frequently used terms from MeSH. If necessary these MeSH terms are cross-referenced to their equivalent term in the *Excerpta Medica* thesaurus, Malimet.

MALIMET

Before proceeding to examples using the *Guide to the Classification and Indexing System* it might be assumed that the thesaurus criteria would be similar to those used in MeSH. However, for *Excerpta Medica*, as has already been stated, medical specialists rather than indexing specialists are employed. Their depth of understanding and their ability to use specific terminology is high; however, their indexing skills will not be those of the Medlars indexers.

To overcome possible shortfalls Malimet (the *Master List of Medical Terms*) was introduced. A computer authority file rather than a thesaurus, Malimet permits the indexer to use free text which is then translated into standardised terminology. Malimet ensures standard American spelling of terms, that all noun forms are singular, that natural word order is maintained, and that the preferred internationally accepted terminology is used. Malimet does this by having four major authority files. These have a quarter of a million preferred terms, slightly more synonyms, the complete classification system on-line, and an additional Emtag item index.

Any term used by the indexer is automatically compared with the files. If it is in the preferred term file, this term will be used to index the article; if not, the synonyms are checked. If it is found here, then the corresponding preferred term is assigned; if not, and it is not being used as a tag, then it is printed out for action. A special editorial committee decides whether or not the term is a synonym, a spelling error, or a new term to be added to the file. This ensures that the indexing is updated as medical terminology changes. For example, if a synonym is being used more frequently than the listed preferred term then the synonym will become the preferred term.

Malimet is available on microfiche though it cannot be said to be easy to use. Preferred terms should always be used in searching specific concepts. The microfiche shows the synonym listed under each preferred term with a frequency of use count. Some of the synonynms are asterisked. This indicates that previously the synonym was a preferred term. This is an historical note equivalent to those used in MeSH (see MeSH example, **Gamma Globulins**), therefore retrospective searching should use the asterisked preferred term.

If a copy of the microfiche is available, look at it and make up you own mind as to its usefulness. Compare it with the information given for terms in MeSH. Unlike MeSH, users are not encouraged to use the microfiche Malimet. Use of the *Guide to the Subject Index Terminology* is however important.

GUIDE TO THE SUBJECT INDEX TERMINOLOGY

This is printed on the blue pages in the *Guide to the Classification and Indexing System* and comprises an alphabetical listing of concepts covered by the abstract journals. There are approximately 5,000 biomedical terms derived from the most frequently used Malimet and MeSH terms. Using this guide requires the user to think of broad concepts. From these concepts one is guided to the most appropriate *Excerpta Medica* section in which a detailed search can begin. The index is therefore not attempting to be specific — it would indeed be difficult with only 5,000 concepts listed — but it is a guide to the abstract journals.

With the same examples we used for MeSH, look up **Phenothiazine Tranquilizers**. It is perhaps not surprising that there is no entry. Using the broader term **Tranquilizer** the entry reads as shown in Figure 21. This is enough information to guide the user to the most appropriate sections. The bold print volumes are the most important.

If a search requires consideration of a number of concepts, then each can be checked in the same way and sections in common (if any) can be found.

---

tranquilizer   24, 30, **32, 37** 38
   major tranquilizer
      use neuroleptic agent 24, 30, **32,**
                              37, 38

Figure 21. From the guide to the subject index terminology on the blue pages of the *Guide to the Classification and Indexing System*

EXCERPTA MEDICA CLASSIFICATION SYSTEM (EMCLAS)

Each of the sections which make up *Excerpta Medica* has its own hierarchical classification system. Each hierarchy enables the user to search an entire category of concepts which may correspond to a number of Malimet preferred terms. This will yield a higher number of references than searching on a broad indexing term.

With the example **Tranquilizers**, consider a search for articles on the *use of* tranquilizers. The numbers to the right of the search term on the blue pages of the *Guide* refer the searcher first to sections 32 and 37. To check quickly what these are, and if one is more likely to be relevant than the other, open out the flap on the back cover of the *Guide to the Classification and Indexing System*. 32 is psychiatry, 37 is drug literature index. Assume that it is the use in psychiatry we are interested in. Turn to section 32 on the beige pages *Excerpta Medica* Classification System. Here you will see a detailed structure following a brief introduction to the section (see Figure 22). The

Psychiatry

This abstract journal covers all aspects of the work and training of the psychiatrist.

The information begins with chapters on medical psychology, mental tests, psychophysiology, psycho-chemistry, genetics and endocrinology. It continues with separate chapters for each type of mental illness encountered (mental deficiency, organic brain syndromes, psychoses, neuroses, addiction, suicide, etc.) and each therapeutic approach employed (psychotherapy, psychoanalyses, group therapy, psychopharmacology, convulsive therapy, etc.).

There are also separate chapters for electro-encephalography, sexology, occupational therapy, social psychiatry, child psychiatry, geriatric psychiatry, forensic psychiatry, military psychiatry and other general areas.

Audience: Psychiatrists, therapists, neurologists.

1. HISTORY AND GENERAL ASPECTS
2. MEDICAL PSYCHOLOGY
    2.1. Experimental psychology
    2.2. Thinking and learning
    2.3. Memory
3. MENTAL TESTS
    3.1. Intelligence tests
    3.2. Projective tests
    3.3. Diagnostic tests
4. PSYCHOPHYSIOLOGY
    4.1. Sleeping and dreaming
    4.2. Experimental psychophysiology
    4.3. Conditioning
5. PSYCHOCHEMISTRY
    5.1. Experimental psychochemistry
    5.2. Psychotomimetics
6. ENDOCRINOLOGY
7. ELECTROENCEPHALOGRAPHY
8. GENERAL PSYCHOPATHOLOGY
9. GENETICS
10. MENTAL DEFICIENCY
    10.1. Education and etiology
    10.2. Mental health services
    10.3. Mongolism
11. ORGANIC BRAIN SYNDROMES
    11.1. Symptomatic psychosis
    11.2. Dementia
    11.3. Brain tumors
12. PSYCHOSIS
    12.1. Schizophrenia
    12.2. Depression and mania
13. NEUROSIS
14. PSYCHOSOMATIC MEDICINE
15. SEXOLOGY
    15.1. Sexual behavior
    15.2. Sexual deviation
    15.3. Birth control
16. INTOXICATION
    16.1. Incidence
    16.2. Treatment
17. ADDICTION
    17.1. Incidence
    17.2. Etiology
    17.3. Treatment
18. ALCOHOLISM
    18.1. Incidence
    18.2. Treatment
    18.3. Delirium tremens
19. PSYCHOTHERAPY
    19.1. Behavior therapy
20. PSYCHOANALYSIS
    20.1. Psychoanalytic treatment
21. GROUP THERAPY
    21.1. Group dynamics
    21.2. Group psychotherapy
    21.3. Family therapy
22. HYPNOSIS
23. PSYCHOPHARMACOLOGY
    23.1. Experimental psycho-pharmacology
    23.2. Drug treatment
    23.3. Adverse drug reactions
24. CONVULSIVE TREATMENT
25. SURGICAL TREATMENT
26. UNCLASSIFIED TREATMENT
27. OCCUPATIONAL THERAPY AND REHABILITATION
28. SOCIAL PSYCHIATRY
    28.1. Mental health
    28.2. Mental hospital
29. CHILD PSYCHIATRY
    29.1. Education
    29.2. Behavior disorders and neurosis
    29.3. Psychosis
30. ADOLESCENCE
    30.1. Development
    30.2. Student
31. GERIATRIC PSYCHIATRY
32. SUICIDE
    32.1. Epidemiology
    32.2. Prevention
    32.3. Psychodynamics
33. FORENSIC PSYCHIATRY
    33.1. Law and court
    33.2. Juvenile delinquency
34. MILITARY PSYCHIATRY
    34.1. Aviation and space flight
35. PREVENTIVE MENTAL HYGIENE
36. EDUCATION AND TRAINING

Figure 22. From the beige pages of the *Guide to the Classification and Indexing System*

introduction states what is covered by *Abstract Journal* (32) and who the intended audience are (in this case they are psychiatrists, therapists and neurologists). Looking through the terms in the classification system, **Tranquilizer** as a heading does not appear anywhere in the classification system. However Chapter 23 is entitled Psychopharmacology, and subdivision 23.2 is Drug Treatment. The codes are particularly useful for on-line searching, which will be discussed in a future volume.

Before moving onto searching in the *Abstract Journals* themselves, there are other sections in the *Guide* which need consideration.

THE INDEX TO EMCLAS

The index is used mainly for on-line searching. However with the term **Tranquilizer** we can find at which chapter in the mentioned sections we are likely to retrieve articles on this topic. The index is arranged alphabetically and in the 1983 edition of the *Guide* it is found on the green pages (see Figure 23). The term **Tranquilizers** will be found in four sections (24, 30, 37 and 38). This does not mean that relevant articles are not in

---

Tranquilizers
 see also under the specific drugs
 and drug groups
 24.6.12 (pharmacology)
 30.6.1
 37.3.5
 38.8 (major tranquilizers)

Figure 23. From the green pages of the *Guide to the Classification and Indexing System*

---

section 32 only that the *term* does not appear. Look up 30.6.1 on the beige pages (see Figure 24). **Tranquilizers** as a psychotropic agent in general pharmacology can be found. You can check the other sections mentioned to check the various emphases — e.g. 37.3.5 shows tranquilizers as psychotropic agents in the drug literature index.

THE INDEX TO EMTAGS

Tags have been mentioned in Section 1 on Medlars. They are

Pharmacology

Section 30 contains an introductory chapter dealing with general problems such as pharmacokinetics, drug receptor interactions, bioassays and metabolism. A number of separate chapters are devoted to drugs affecting particular organs or organ systems or to drugs exerting a particular type of action, including the autonomic nervous system, the motor system, psychotropic and neurotropic drugs, anesthetics, analgesics, antiinflammatory agents, the cardiovascular system, the digestive system, the endocrine system, antineoplastic agents and several others.

A number of other chapters cover topics such as diagnostic agents, disinfectants, immunologic agents, anticaries agents, drug vehicles and additives.

Starting in 1983, most of the information on pesticides, phytocides and toxic substances will be transferred to a new section (no. 52) on Toxicology.

This section is an essential reference and alerting tool for keeping up to date with advances across a broad spectrum of interest in pharmacology.

Audience: Experimental and clinical pharmacologists and clinical pharmacists in hospitals, industry, universities and general practice.

1. GENERAL ASPECTS
    1.1. History
    1.2. Pharmacokinetics
        1.2.1. Drug metabolism
    1.3. Drug receptor interactions
    1.4. Bioassays and biostatistics
    1.5. Techniques and apparatus
    1.6. Metabolism
        1.6.1. Protein and nucleic acid metabolism
        1.6.2. Carbohydrate and lipid metabolism
        1.6.3. Enzymes
    1.7. Pharmacogenetics
2. AUTONOMIC NERVOUS SYSTEM
    2.1. Cholinergic system
        2.1.1. Cholinergics (parasympathomimetics)
        2.1.2. Anticholinergics (parasympatholytics)
        2.1.3. Cholinesterase inhibitors
        2.1.4. Cholinesterase reactivators
    2.2. Adrenergic system
        2.2.1. alpha-Adrenergic stimulants
        2.2.2. alpha-Adrenergic blockers
        2.2.3. beta-Adrenergic stimulants
        2.2.4. beta-Adrenergic blockers
        2.2.5. Pseudoadrenergic stimulants
        2.2.6. Adrenergic neuron blockers
    2.3. Agents affecting ganglia
3. MOTOR SYSTEM
    3.1. Antiparkinson agents
    3.2. Tremorigenic agents
    3.3. Central acting muscle relaxants
    3.4. Neuromuscular blockers
4. ANESTHETICS
    4.1. General anesthetics
    4.2. Anesthetic premedication
    4.3. Local anesthetics
5. CENTRAL DEPRESSANTS
    5.1. Hypnotic sedatives
    5.2. Antiepileptics
6. PSYCHOTROPIC AND NEUROTROPIC AGENTS
    6.1. Tranquilizers
    6.2. Neuroleptics
    6.3. Antidepressants
        6.3.1. Thymoleptics
        6.3.2. MAO inhibitors
    6.4. Psychostimulants
    6.5. Psychotomimetics
    6.6. Neurotransmitters
    6.7. Analeptic agents
7. ANOREXIANTS
8. ANALGESICS AND ANTIINFLAMMATORY AGENTS
    8.1. Narcotic analgesics and antagonists
    8.2. Antipyretic analgesics
9. ANTISPASMODICS; AGENTS AFFECTING SMOOTH MUSCLE
10. AUTACOIDS
    10.1. Histamine and antagonists
        10.1.1. Histamine and analogs
        10.1.2. Antihistamines
    10.2. Serotonin and antagonists
        10.2.1. Serotonin and analogs
        10.2.2. Serotonin antagonists
    10.3. Kinins and antagonists
11. CARDIOVASCULAR SYSTEM
    11.1. Cardiac glycosides
    11.2. Antiarrhythmic and arrhythmia inducing agents
    11.3. Antihypertensive agents
    11.4. Pressor agents
    11.5. Coronary dilators
    11.6. Peripheral vasoactive agents
    11.7. Agents affecting lipid metabolism
12. EMETICS AND ANTIEMETICS
    12.1. Antiemetics
    12.2. Emetics
13. AGENTS AFFECTING BODY FLUID VOLUME AND COMPOSITION
    13.1. Plasma volume expanders
    13.2. Diuretics
14. HEMOPOIETIC AND RETICULOENDOTHELIAL SYSTEM
    14.1. Iron containing substances
    14.2. Trace elements
    14.3. Vitamins
15. HEMOSTASIS
    15.1. Vitamin K group
    15.2. Anticoagulants
    15.3. Fibrinolytics and antifibrinolytics
16. RESPIRATORY SYSTEM
    16.1. Bronchodilators
    16.2. Expectorants
    16.3. Respiratory mucolytics
    16.4. Antitussives
17. DIGESTIVE SYSTEM

Figure 24. From the beige pages of the *Guide to the Classification and Indexing System*

used to index broad or secondary concepts — e.g. the route of administration, the experimental animal, the organ system affected, etc. Although these terms are included on the blue pages, the *Guide* also lists them all on the yellow pages (starting at p.205 of the 1983 edition). Terms introduced since March 1978 are given one asterisk; those introduced since January 1983 have two asterisks. Each tag has a scope note to explain its use. Codes are given to each tag for on-line searching.

CLASS A AND B TERMS

In Medlars there are major and minor descriptors. In *Excerpta Medica* their equivalents are A and B terms. Only class A terms, the major descriptors, are used as entry points in the printed subject indices of the *Abstract Journals*. The distinction is not usually relevant for on-line searching. If there is additional information which the indexer wishes to use, then it can be added as secondary terms. They are free text, not checked against Malimet, and can be regarded as 'text-enrichers'.

The *Guide* should be used whenever a search in a new subject area is started. The subject index guides the user to the appropriate section of *Excerpta Medica*; the classification scheme guides the user to the appropriate chapters within the section; and the codes are very useful for on-line searching, as well as for gathering related abstracts together in the *Abstract Journals* (see Figure 24).

PROBLEMS WITH THE *GUIDE*

SPELLING

As with Medlars, American spelling is used which can be a problem for English spellers; for example in alphabetisation. If you look up **Oestrogen Therapy** in the subject index, there is no cross-reference to the preferred term **Estrogen.**

SPECIFICITY OF TERMS

With only 5,000 terms in the subject index the user has to broaden the search, and from this broad term redefine it when searching the individual sections of *Excerpta Medica*.

On the other hand, the *Guide* uses jargon which may be unfamiliar to the new user. Many may consider it best to use only the flap on the inside back cover. This gives the titles of each of the sections, and from these headings, the average reader may consider the next step is the section itself.

WORD FORMS

Excerpta Medica, like Medlars, uses Anglo-Saxon, Greek and Latin terminology, particularly with organs such as the kidney. In this case the problem is not as great as for MeSH where terms can be lost altogether, but it can still be confusing. Look up **Nephropathy** on the blue pages (Figure 25). There is a 'use' reference to **Kidney Disease**, but the searcher does not need to turn to K to find the appropriate sections as they are specified at the 'see' reference. It does mean, however, that care will be needed when searching.

---

nephropathy
use kidney disease   5, 6, 7, 20, **28**

Figure 25. From the blue pages of the *Guide to the Classification and Indexing System*

AMERICAN TERMINOLOGY

Under the term **Cot Death** there is a 'use sudden infant death', with an appropriate section.

TERM INVERSION

This should not be the problem it was with MeSH where some terms were in natural word order and others were inverted. The rule with *Excerpta Medica* is to use natural word order.

Generally the problems are less obvious than for *Index Medicus* and most are overcome when using the actual sections. We will look again at the *Guide* in a future volume which considers on-line searching.

THE INDIVIDUAL SECTIONS

Each section has a number of issues which are published periodically throughout the year. Each issue begins with the classification system as shown in the *Guide* and gives an example of an entry, with explanation. Following this come the abstracts in classification number order. Within the chapters referring to the major divisions of the classification system come individual abstracts. The abstracts, following assignment to chapters, are numbered sequentially with number 1 appearing in the first issue of the year.

The most important section is the subject index. This is computer-generated but without using secondary terms as lead-ins. This keeps the size of the index within a reasonable limit. Each major descriptor appears in the index followed by other major descriptors, minor descriptors and check tags. Finally, each entry is given a number referring to the abstract or abstracts in which the term can be found.

Look up **Chlorpromazine** in section 32, volume 50, issue 8 (1984) (see Figure 26). Two abstracts are mentioned. The first is

---

chlorpromazine, adenosine triphosphate, promazine, promethazine, trifluoperazine, triflupromazine, drug binding, micellar solubilization, 2455
 - fluphenazine, haloperidol, mania, schizophrenia, thioridazine, neuroleptic agent, dosing practice, 110 patients, 2481

Figure 26. From section 32, volume 50, issue 8 of *Excerpta Medica*

---

the number 2455. This is the abstract number and can be found in this particular issue. This gives some information as to the relevance of the abstract to the work being carried out. The second item shows the tag's 'dosing practice' and 110 patients which again enriches the index entry.

THE AUTHOR INDEX

If the author is known, then an article can be traced using the author index. All authors cited in the abstract reference whether the first named or not, appear in the author index. Where more than three authors appear, then only the first three are named.

THE ABSTRACT

Following the abstract number is the title, the authors (up to three), and the full bibliographic citation. This is followed by the abstract which can be quite lengthy and detailed (see Figure 27). As an abstract may take some time to produce, and as an article abstracted for one section may have been previously abstracted for another section, the time-lag between publication of an article in a primary journal and its inclusion as an abstract in an *EM* section can be considerable.

2455. Behavior of ATP toward phenothiazine drugs - Gasco M.R., Carlotti M.E. and Trotta M. - Istituto di Chimica Farmaceutica e Tossicologica, Universita di Torino, 10125 Torino ITA - *J. PHARM. SCI.* 1984 73/5 (662–666)

The tricyclic amines promazine, promethazine, chlorpromazine, triflupromazine, and trifluperazine form solid ion pairs with ATP in a 1:2 molar ratio. There is a good correlation between the measured K(sp) and the apparent diffusion constants of the ion pairs with the critical micelle concentration (CMC) of the corresponding phenothiazines. Solid ion pairs are solubilized by phenothiazine micelles; the binding constants of ATP to drug micelles are calculated from solubility data at 25°C and can be related to the CMC of the phenothiazines.

Figure 27. From section 32, volume 50, issue 8, of *Excerpta Medica*

CUMULATED YEARLY *EXCERPTA MEDICA*

This has a similar layout to the individual sections. The classification system has in addition to headings, page numbers where that section first appears within the cumulation. Using section 32, chapter 12, Psychosis begins on p.18 of issue 1, on p.75 of issue 2, p.128 of issue 3, etc. (see Figure 28). Although this is explained in the text of the 'How to use' section, it is not immediately clear from the table itself. The numbering of the abstracts flows from 1 to the end, but the classification scheme recurs with each issue.

CONTENTS
1. HISTORY AND GENERAL ASPECTS 1, -, -, 163, 217, 271, 323, 375, 431, 487.
2. MEDICAL PSYCHOLOGY 1, 55, 109, 163, 217, 271, 323, 375, 431, 487.
  2.1. Experimental psychology 3, -, 111, 164, 219, 273, 324, 377, 432, -.
  2.2. Thinking and learning 3, 56, 111, 164, 219, -, -, 377. -, 489.
  2.3. Memory 3, 56, 112, 164, 219, 274, 325, 377, -, 490.
3. MENTAL TESTS 4, 57, 112, 165, 220, 274, 325, 378, 432, 490.
  3.1. Intelligence tests 4, -, -, 165, -, -, 325, -, 433, 491.
  3.2. Projective tests -, -, -, -, -, -, -, 379, -, 491.
  3.3. Diagnostic tests 4, 57, 113, 165, 221, 275, 325, 379, 433, 492.
4. PSYCHOPHYSIOLOGY 6, 59, 114, 166, 223, 277, 327, 380, 434, 493.
  4.1. Sleeping and dreaming 7, 60, 114, 167, 223, 277, 327, 380, 435, 494.
  4.2. Experimental psychophysiology 7, 61, 115, 167, 224, 278, 327, -, 436, 495.
  4.3. Conditioning -, 61, 116, 168, 224, 278, 328, 382, -, 496.
5. PSYCHOCHEMISTRY 7, 61, 116, 168, 225, 278, 328, 382, 436, 497.
  5.1. Experimental psychochemistry 10, 64, 119, 171, 227, 280, -, 385, 439, -.
  5.2. Psychotomimetics -, 64. -, -, -, -, -, -, -, -.
6. ENDOCRINOLOGY 11, 65, 119, 172, 228, 281, 329, 385, 440, 497.
7. ELECTROENCEPHALOGRAPHY 12, 67, 121, 173, 229, 282, 329, 387, 442, 498.
8. GENERAL PSYCHOPATHOLOGY 12, 69, 122, 175, 231, 282, 330, 387, 442, 499.
9. GENETICS 14, 70, 123, 175, 232, 284, 332, 389, 443, 501.
10. MENTAL DEFICIENCY 14, 71, 123, 175, 232, 284, 332, 389, 443, 501.
  10.1. Education and etiology 15, 72, 123, 176, 233, 285, 332, 389, 444, 501.
  10.2. Mental health services 15, 72, -, -, -, -, 333, 389, -, 502.
  10.3. Mongolism 15, 73, 123, 177, -, 285, 333, 390, 444, 502.
11. ORGANIC BRAIN SYNDROMES 16, 73, 124, 177, 234, 286, 333, 391, 444, 502.
  11.1. Symptomatic psychosis 16, 73, 125, 177, 234, 287, 335, 391, 445, 502.
  11.2. Dementia 17, 74, 126, 178, 235, 287, 355, 391, 445, 503.
  11.3. Brain tumors -, 75, -, -, -, -, -, 392, -, 504.
12. PSYCHOSIS 18, 75, 128, 178, 235, 287, 336, 392, 447, 504.
  12.1. Schizophrenia 18, 75, 128, 179, 235, 290, 337, 393, 447, 504.
  12.2. Depression and mania 19, 76, 128, 179, 237, 290, 338, 395, 449, 506.
13. NEUROSIS 21, 77, 130, 181, 239, 292, 340, 396, 450, 507.
14. PSYCHOSOMATIC MEDICINE 22, 77, 131, 181, 239, 292, 341, 396, 450, 509.
15. SEXOLOGY 24, 80, 132, 182, 241, 294, 344, 399, 452, 512.
  15.1. Sexual behavior 25, 80, 132, 183, 242, 294, 344, 400, 453, 513.
  15.2. Sexual deviation 25, 80, 132, 183, 242, 294, -, 400, 453, 513.
  15.3. Birth control 26, -, 133, 184, -, -, 345, 401. -, -.
16. INTOXICATION 26, 80, 133, 184, -, 295, 345, 402, 453, 514.
  16.1. Incidence 26, 80, 133, 184, -, 295, 345, 402, 453, 514.
  16.2. Treatment -, 82, -, 185, -, -, -, -, 402, 454, 514.
17. ADDICTION 27, 82, 133, 185, 242, 296, 346, 402, 454, 515.
  17.1. Incidence 27, 82, -, 185, -, 296, 346, 402, 455, 516.
  17.2. Etiology 27, 83, 133, -, 242, 297, -, 402, 455, -.
  17.3. Treatment 28, 83, 134, 186, 242, 297, 346, 403, 455, 516.
18. ALCOHOLISM 29, 84, 135, 186, 243, 298, 347, 403, 456, 517.
  18.1. Incidence 29, 85, 135, 188, 244, 300, 348, 404, 457, 519.
  18.2. Treatment 30, 87, 136, 190, 245, 300, 349, 406, 458, 519.
  18.3. Delirium tremens -, -, 137, -, -, -, -, -, -, 520.
19. PSYCHOTHERAPY 31, 88, 138, 191, 245, 301, 349, 406, 459, 520.
  19.1. Behavior therapy 32, 89, 139, 191, 248, 302, 351, 407, 459, 521.
20. PSYCHOANALYSIS 33, 90, 141, 192, 250, 304, 353, 408, 461, 523.
  20.1. Psychoanalytic treatment 33, 91, -, -, 250, 305, 353, 409, 461, -.
21. GROUP THERAPY 33, -, 142, 192, 251, 305, 353, 409, 462, 523.
  21.1. Group dynamics -, -, 142, -, 251, -, -, -, -, 523.
  21.2. Group psychotherapy 34, -, -, 193, 251, 305, 353, 409, -, -.
  21.3. Family therapy 34, -, 142, 193, 252, 305, -, 410, 462, -.
22. HYPNOSIS 34, 91, 142, 193, 253, 306, 353, 411, 462, 524.

Figure 28. From section 32, Cumulated *Excerpta Medica*

The subject index is cumulated so that if you look up **Chlorpromazine**, there are some 20 references each with its associated minor descriptors and tags, and each with an abstract number (see Figure 29).

chlorpromazine, acute psychosis, schizophrenia, sulpiride, double blind procedure, drug efficacy, drug tolerance, comparison in 61 cases, 61 patients, 1946
- adrenergic receptor, brain cortex, imipramine, 4 aminoclonidine h 3, alpha 2 adrenergic receptor, beta adrenergic receptor, depression, dihydroalprenolol h 3, drug mixture, rat, 226
- adverse drug reaction, brain, flavine adenine nucleotide, riboflavin deficiency, rat, 2989
- alcohol dehydrogenase liver level, aldehyde dehydrogenase, enzyme inhibition, in vitro study, mouse, 1939
- amitriptyline, glucuronide, imipramine, mass spectrometry, patient, rabbit, 1234
- anorexia nervosa, growth hormone, levodopa, prolactin, 6 female patients, 3129
- behavior, memory, motor activity, state dependent learning, rat, 908
- blood pressure, cigarette smoking, pharmacokinetics, sleep, drug interaction, hypotension, metabolism, sleepiness, 270
- brain, cholinesterase blocking agent, cholinesterase, insecticide agent, mevinphos, physostigmine, azinphos, carbaryl, dimpylate, drug interaction, haloperidol, heart muscle, kidney, liver, lung, muscle, rat, 895
- chlordiazepoxide, cocaine, food intake, instrumental conditioning, behavior, reinforcement, squirrel monkey, 2259
- chlorpromazine sulfoxide, pharmacokinetics, radioimmunoassay, drug blood level, volunteer, 2261
- clozapine, desipramine, dopamine receptor, extrapyramidal symptom, haloperidol, neuroleptic agent, promethazine, sulpiride, 4 aminobutyric acid, rat, 1244
- dopamine release, prolactin blood level, schizophrenia, human, 2274
- erythrocyte, imipramine, lithium, phosphatidylethanolamine methyltransferase, ghost cell, human, 3303
- learning disorder, teratogenicity, newborn, rat, 2618
- neuroleptic agent, prolactin blood level, schizophrenia, clinical study, serum, 10 females, 11 males, 21 patients, 1953
- schizophrenia, serotonin, thrombocyte, 19 patients, 900
- schizophrenia, outpatient, recurrence risk, 268

Figure 29. From the Cumulated *Excerpta Medica*, subject index

There is a cumulated author index covering the full year.

Searching in *Excerpta Medica*

Consider the use of **ranitidine** as an H_2-receptor blocking agent. First check in the subject index of the *Guide to the Classification System*. Not surprisingly, there is no entry. If we know nothing more about the drug we can go to **Drug Treatment**, again in the subject index (see Figure 30). This guides the user to pharmacotherapy, but you are given sections 30 and 37 on the

---

drug treatment
use pharmacotherapy   30, **37**

Figure 30. From the blue pages of the *Guide to the Classification and Indexing System*

---

back flap. You can now see that section 30 is pharmacology and section 37 is the drug literature index.

If at this point you know that ranitidine is a drug used for treating stomach ulcers, you may wish to look up **Stomach Ulcer** (Figure 31). If you do you will find two sections: 9,

---

stomach ulcer   9, **48**

Figure 31. From the blue pages of the *Guide to the Classification and Indexing System*

which is Surgery, and **48** which is Gastroenterology. As drug treatment is more likely with gastroenterology you can check the beige pages of the *Guide* to look at the classification system. This doesn't appear particularly helpful so move straight to sections 48 and 30 to see if relevant references are available.

Ranitidine is cited in 17 cases in section 48 of the cumulated *EM*, volume 25, 1984 (Figure 32). Some of these appear relevant, though many compare its activity with that of cimetidine. In section 30, Pharmacology, there are four references in cumulated *EM*, volume 59, 1984, many of which are the same. As ranitidine was marketed three or four years ago, it may not be surprising that articles on treatment will have diminished.

---

ranitidine, albumin cr 51, alpha 1 antitrypsin, menetrier disease, patient of 37, 950
  - antihistaminic agent, cimetidine, drug interaction, liver, cytochrome p450, drug elimination, glucuronidation, pharmacokinetics, 955
  - burimamide, cimetidine, histamine h2 receptor antagonist, imidazole, oxmetidine, thrombocyte aggregation, adenosine diphosphate, collagen, in vitro study, 680

  - chronic kidney failure, duodenum ulcer, pharmacokinetics, drug blood level, drug elimination, patient, 1823
  - cigarette smoking, cimetidine, duodenum ulcer, oxmetidine, endoscopy, recurrence risk, 135 patients, 1821
  - cimetidine, stomach ulcer, antacid agent, endoscopy, pain, therapy, 71 outpatients, 405
  - cimetidine, jejunum ulcer, zollinger ellison syndrome, case report, 402
  - cimetidine, stomach ulcer, therapy, comparison in 44 cases, 44 outpatients, double blind trial, 1535
  - cimetidine, stomach acid, stomach hypersecretion, adverse drug reaction, androgen antiserum, breast, 2587
  - cimetidine, zollinger ellison syndrome, endoscopy, stomach ph, 24 hour ph measurement, 22
  - drug absorption, drug interaction, hypnotic agent, midazolam, bioavailability, volunteer, 1453
  - duodenum ulcer, stomach acid secretion, stomach ulcer, wound healing, double blind procedure, endoscopy, 48 patients, 1820
  - electron microscopy, omeprazole, stomach acid secretion, stomach biopsy, stomach fistula, stomach parietal cell, dog, 2303
  - esophagitis, gastrin, gastroesophageal reflux, stomach emptying, technetium sulfur colloid tc 99m, double blind procedure, placebo, radioimmunoassay, 73 patients, 1505
  - kidney failure, pharmacokinetics, bioavailability, creatinine clearance, 2661
  - metoclopramide, reflux esophagitis, endoscopy, histology, therapy, 45 patients, 67
  - reflux esophagitis, esophagoscopy, trial, double blind trial, 1518
  - stomach ulcer, cytochrome p450, drug interaction, liver, survey, 33 references, 690

Figure 32. From section 48, volume 25, Cumulated *Excerpta Medica*

Conclusion

I have described the use of two of the most commonly used sources of medical information. Between them, *Index Medicus* and *Excerpta Medica* cover the vast majority of published literature in the medical sciences. Both have problems with their use and to some extent have attempted to overcome them by means of additional guides and aids. If the inherent problems of language and term format are understood, the use of both sources will be more rewarding and effective.

The use of these sources will be discussed in the forthcoming volume *How to Use Biological Abstracts, Chemical Abstracts and Psychological Abstracts*. The third volume in the series, *How to Search the Medical Sources* will consider search strategies and techniques. This will take a specific topic and discuss the relative merits of searching using the sources previously discussed. Criteria for the selection of on-line sources versus the printed version will also be included.

Subject index

This is an Index to main topics of interest, there is a separate index of examples.

A and B terms 47
Abstracts 49
Allowable categories in *Index Medicus* 24
Alphabetisation 28, 47
Anglo-American Spelling 27, 47
Annotated MeSH 9, 11
Author Index 33, 49

Bibliography of Medical Reviews 32
Bibliographies, recurring 3
Blaise 4

Check Tags 20, 49
Citation types 20
Classification System 43
Combination therapy (Treatment in MeSH) 18
Compilation of *Index Medicus*, by computer 3
Compound terms 15, 24-5
Controlled vocabulary 5
Cumulated *Excerpta Medica* 50
Cumulated *Index Medicus* 31

Data Form Abbreviations 21

Data-Star 4
Dialog, *see* Lockheed, Dialog

Emclas 43
  Index 45
Emtags 45
  Index 45
Entry Terms 21
Entry Versions 21
Excerpta Medica 35
  Format 40

Fixed text *see* controlled vocabulary 6

Geographic Headings 20
Guide to the Classification and Indexing System of *Excerpta Medica* 42
Guide to the Subject Index Terminology 42

Headings in *Index Medicus* 5
  Assignment 5

Index Medicus 3, 31
  Cumulated 31

Monthly   33
Index to Dental Literature   3, 4
Indexing of Medlars   5
   Decentralisation   5
   Depth   5
International Nursing Index   3, 4

Journal Coverage, *see* List of Journals Indexed

Language problems   25, 26, 48
List of Journals Indexed (IM)
   Index Medicus   31
   Excerpta Medica   38
Lockheed Dialog   4

Main Headings of *Index Medicus*   20
Major descriptors   19
Malimet   41
Medlars
   as a bi product   3
   history   4
Medlars online *see* Medline   4
Medline   4
MeSH   7
MeSH Supplementary Chemical Records   16
   MeSH, Public *see* Public MeSH
   MeSH, Annotated *see* Annotated MeSH
   MeSH, Permuted *see* Permuted MeSH
Minor descriptors   21

National Library of Medicine   4
NLM *see* National Library of Medicine
Non-MeSH   20

Permuted MeSH   13-15
Pre-coordinated headings   28
Primary Journals   5

Public MeSH   7

Retrospective searches   9
   from *Index Medicus*   4
Registry numbers   16
Reviews   32
Rush journals   5

Searching
   Excerpta Medica   53
   Index Medicus   7
Secondary Journals   5
"See Under" terms   8
Selective indexing   5
Specificity of terms   9
   in *Excerpta Medica*   47
Subject Index of *Excerpta Medica*   52
Subheadings in *Index Medicus*   24
Supplementary Chemical Records *see* MeSH Supplementary Chemical Records
Synonyms   29
   approach using *Index Medicus*   29
   approach using *Excerpta Medica see* Malimet   4

Tags, Check *see* Check Tags
Term inversion *see also* Compound terms   28, 48
Topical Subheadings with Scope Notes and Allowable Categories   23
Tree Codes   9
Tree Structures   11-13

Word forms
   problems in *Index Medicus*   25
   problems in *Excerpta Medica*   48

"XU" terms   8

Index of examples

Alta 29
Agammaglobulinemia 9
AIDS 19
3-Aminopropionic Acid 28
Animal 20
Arm 25
Arm Injuries 25
Amebiasis 27
Amobarbital 27
Amoebiasis 27
Amylobarbital 27

Background Radiation 28
Berner, B. D. 33
Bibliography 32
Bronchography 21

Canogenin Thevetoside 13
Cardiac Glycosides 13
Case Reports 20
CAT 29
Chlorpromazine 49–52
Convalleria Glycosides 13
Cot Death 27, 48
Crib Death 27

DELTA 29
Dental Service, Hospital 11
Diagnosis, Respiratory System 21
Digitalis Glycosides 13

Diaper Rash 27
Drug Treatment 53

Echinococcosis, Pulmonary 15
Embolism, Air 28
EMI 29
Eng. Abstr. 33
Estrogen 27, 47

Female 20
Forms and Records Control,
    Growth and Embryonic
    Development 28
Furans 32, 33, 34

Gamma Globulins 9–11, 20, 25, 42
Globulin Deficiency 9

Head 25
Head Injuries 25
Hospital Dental Service 11
Human 20
Hydatid Cyst Pulmonary 15

JAMA 31–32, 38

Kidney 25
    Cortex 25, 26

Disease 25, 26, 48

Lactate Dehydrogenase 21
Leg 25
Leg Injuries 25

Mercaptopropionic Acid 28
Methyl Atropine *see* Methylatropine
Methylatropine 16-17

Napkin Rash 27
Nappy Rash 27
Necrosis 25
Nephrectomy 25
Nephritis 25
Nephropathy 48
Nephrosclerosis 25

Oestrogen 27
   Therapy 47

P-Aminosalicylic Acid 28
Paraquat 24
Pharmacodynamics 32
Phenothiazine Tranquilizers 7-9, 43

Prenatal Explosure, Delayed Effects 28
Protein Methyltransferase III 28
Protein Methyltransferases 28
Protein O-Methyltransferase 28
Psychiatry 44
   Military 21-22
Pulmonary 13-15

Rachitis 21
Radiation, Background 28
Ranitidine 53-54
Renal Osteodystrophy 25
   Circulation 25
Respiratory Sounds 21
Respiratory System 21
ROAP 18

SID 27
Stomach Ulcer 53
Sudden Infant Death 27

Therapeutic Use 32
Tomography, X-Ray Computed 29
Tranquilizers 43-46
Tuberculosis in Childhood 28

Vaccines 25